The Quickening Pulse

The Quickening Pulse

Books 1–5

to accompany
Excellence in English Books 1–5

The Quickening Pulse

Book 2

Selected by D J Brindley

HODDER AND STOUGHTON
LONDON SYDNEY AUCKLAND TORONTO

I should like to thank my wife for her devoted help in the preparation of this book.

1979 DJB

British Library Cataloguing in Publication Data

The quickening pulse.
Book 2
1. Short stories, English
I. Brindley, David James
823'.9'1FS PR1309.S5

ISBN 0 340 23494 6

First published 1979

Fourth impression 1985

Printed and bound in Great Britain for
Hodder and Stoughton Educational,
a division of Hodder and Stoughton Ltd,
Mill Road, Dunton Green, Sevenoaks, Kent,
by Page Bros (Norwich) Ltd

Contents

Charles *by Shirley Jackson*

The day Laurie started kindergarten he renounced corduroy overalls with bibs and began wearing blue jeans with a belt; I watched him go off the first morning with the older girl next door, seeing clearly that an era of my life was ended, my sweet-voiced nursery-school tot replaced by a long-trousered, swaggering character who forgot to stop at the corner and wave goodbye to me.

He came home the same way, the front door slamming open, his cap on the floor,and the voice suddenly became raucous shouting, 'Isn't anybody *here*?'

At lunch he spoke insolently to his father, spilled Jannie's milk and remarked that his teacher said that we were not to take the name of the Lord in vain.

'How was school today?' I asked, elaborately casual.

'All right,' he said.

'Did you learn anything?' his father asked.

Laurie regarded his father coldly. 'I didn't learn nothing,' he said.

'Anything,' I said. 'Didn't learn anything.'

'The teacher spanked a boy, though,' Laurie said, addressing his bread and butter. 'For being fresh,' he added with his mouth full.

'What did he do?' I asked. 'Who was it?'

Laurie thought. 'It was Charles,' he said. 'He was fresh. The teacher spanked him and made him stand in a corner. He was awfully fresh.'

'What did he do?' I asked again, but Laurie slid off his chair, took a cookie, and left, while his father was still saying, 'See here, young man.'

The next day Laurie remarked at lunch, as soon as he sat down, 'Well, Charles was bad again today.' He grinned enormously and said, 'Today Charles hit the teacher.'

'Good heavens,' I said, mindful of the Lord's name, 'I suppose he got spanked again?'

'He sure did,' Laurie said. 'Look up,' he said to his father.

'What?' his father said, looking up.

'Look down,' Laurie said. 'Look at my thumb. Gee, you're dumb.' He began to laugh insanely.

'Why did Charles hit the teacher?' I asked quickly.

'Because she tried to make him colour with red crayons,' Laurie said. 'Charles wanted to colour with green crayons so he hit the teacher and she spanked him and said nobody play with Charles but everybody did.'

The third day—it was Wednesday of the first week—Charles bounced a seesaw onto the head of a little girl and made her bleed and the teacher made him stay inside all during recess. Thursday Charles had to stand in a corner during storytime because he kept pounding his feet on the floor. Friday Charles was deprived of blackboard privileges because he threw chalk.

On Saturday I remarked to my husband, 'Do you think kindergarten is too unsettling for Laurie? All this toughness and bad grammar, and this Charles boy sounds like such a bad influence.'

'It'll be all right,' my husband said reassuringly. 'Bound to be people like Charles in the world. Might as well meet them now as later.'

On Monday Laurie came home late, full of news. 'Charles,' he shouted as he came up the hill; I was waiting anxiously on the front steps; 'Charles,' Laurie yelled all the way up the hill, 'Charles was bad again.'

'Come right in,' I said, as soon as he came close enough. 'Lunch is waiting.'

'You know what Charles did?' he demanded, following me through the door. 'Charles yelled so in school they sent a boy in from first grade to tell the teacher she had to make Charles keep quiet, and so Charles had to stay after school. And so all the children stayed to watch him.'

'What did he do?' I asked.

'He just sat there,' Laurie said, climbing into his chair at the table. 'Hi Pop, y'old dust mop.'

'Charles had to stay after school today,' I told my husband. 'Everyone stayed with him.'

'What does this Charles look like?' my husband asked Laurie. 'What's his other name?'

'He's bigger than me,' Laurie said. 'And he doesn't have any rubbers and he doesn't ever wear a jacket.'

Monday night was the first Parent-Teachers meeting, and only the fact that Jannie had a cold kept me from going; I wanted passionately to meet Charles' mother. On Tuesday Laurie remarked suddenly, 'Our teacher had a friend come see her in school today.'

'Charles' mother?' my husband and I asked simultaneously.

'Naaah,' Laurie said scornfully. 'It was a man who came and made us do exercises. Look.' He climbed down from his chair and squatted down and touched his toes. 'Like this,' he said. He got solemnly back into his chair and said, picking up his fork, 'Charles didn't even *do* exercises.'

'That's fine,' I said heartily. 'Didn't Charles want to do exercises?'

'Naaah,' Laurie said. 'Charles was so fresh to the teacher's friend he wasn't *let* do exercises.'

'Fresh again?' I said.

'He kicked the teacher's friend,' Laurie said. 'The teacher's friend told Charles to touch his toes like I just did and Charles kicked him.'

'What are they going to do about Charles, do you suppose?' Laurie's father asked him.

Laurie shrugged elaborately. 'Throw him out of the school, I guess,' he said.

Wednesday and Thursday were routine; Charles yelled during story hour and hit a boy in the stomach and made him cry. On Friday Charles stayed after school again and so did all the other children.

With the third week of kindergarten Charles was an institution in our family; Jannie was being a Charles when she cried all afternoon; Laurie did a Charles when he filled his wagon full of mud and pulled it through the kitchen; even my husband, when he caught his elbow in the telephone cord and pulled telephone, ash tray, and a bowl of flowers off the table, said, after the first minute, 'Looks like Charles.'

During the third and fourth weeks there seemed to be a reformation in Charles; Laurie reported grimly at lunch on Thursday of the third week, 'Charles was so good today the teacher gave him an apple.'

'What?' I said, and my husband added warily, 'You mean Charles?'

'Charles,' Laurie said. 'He gave the crayons around and he picked up the books afterward and the teacher said he was her helper.'

'What happened?' I asked incredulously.

'He was her helper, that's all,' Laurie said, and shrugged.

'Can this be true, about Charles?' I asked my husband that night. 'Can something like this happen?'

'Wait and see,' my husband said cynically. 'When you've got a Charles to deal with, this may mean he's only plotting.'

He seemed to be wrong. For over a week Charles was the teacher's helper; each day he handed things out and he picked things up; no-one had to stay after school.

'The PTA meeting's next week again,' I told my husband one evening. 'I'm going to find Charles' mother there.'

'Ask her what happened to Charles,' my husband said. 'I'd like to know.'

'I'd like to know myself,' I said.

On Friday of that week things were back to normal. 'You know what Charles did today?' Laurie demanded at the lunch table, in a voice slightly awed. 'He told a little girl to say a word and she said it and the teacher washed her mouth out with soap and Charles laughed.'

'What word?' his father asked unwisely, and Laurie said, 'I'll have to whisper it to you, it's so bad.' He got down off his chair and went around to his father. His father bent his head down and Laurie whispered joyfully. His father's eyes widened.

'Did Charles tell the little girl to say *that*?' he asked respectfully.

'She said it *twice*,' Laurie said. 'Charles told her to say it *twice*.'

'What happened to Charles?' my husband asked.

'Nothing,' Laurie said. 'He was passing out the crayons.'

Monday morning Charles abandoned the little girl and said the evil word himself three or four times, getting his mouth washed out with soap each time. He also threw chalk.

My husband came to the door with me that evening as I set out for the PTA meeting. 'Invite her over for a cup of tea after the meeting,' he said. 'I want to get a look at her.'

'If only she's there,' I said prayerfully.

'She'll be there,' my husband said. 'I don't see how they could hold a PTA meeting without Charles' mother.'

At the meeting I sat restlessly, scanning each comfortable matronly face, trying to determine which one hid the secret of Charles. None of them looked to me haggard enough. No-one stood up in the meeting and apologized for the way her son had been acting. No-one mentioned Charles.

After the meeting I identified and sought out Laurie's kindergarten teacher. She had a plate with a cup of tea and a piece of chocolate cake; I had a plate with a cup of tea and a piece of marshmallow cake. We manoeuvred up to one another cautiously and smiled.

'I've been so anxious to meet you,' I said. 'I'm Laurie's mother.'

'We're all so interested in Laurie,' she said.

'Well, he certainly likes kindergarten,' I said. 'He talks about it all the time.'

'We had a little trouble adjusting, the first week or so,' she said primly, 'but now he's a fine little helper. With lapses, of course.'

'Laurie usually adjusts very quickly,' I said. 'I suppose this time it's Charles' influence.'

'Charles?'

'Yes,' I said, laughing, 'you must have your hands full in that kindergarten, with Charles.'

'Charles?' she said. 'We don't have any Charles in the kindergarten.'

Hoarse Chestnuts *by D J Brindley*

'Every time I come into this room you're making a noise! I've had enough of it. This class is always causing trouble. No, don't start making excuses, I don't want to hear any more. It's about time you learnt to behave decently when a teacher's out of the room. You there! Pay attention! And don't smirk when I talk to you—your impudence has gone beyond a joke. Why were you out of your desk, anyway? And what's that you've got in your hand?'

It was Egghead again—he always caught me doing something odd. I suddenly realised that I'd been standing in the middle of the room and shouting at the top of my voice, swinging my six foot string of horse chestnuts: all carefully pierced and threaded (after having been dipped in vinegar to harden them), ready to battle against any presumptuous rivals from 3A. It was the height of the season, and the craze for conker-fights had spread like an epidemic around the school. I had a marvellous array: large and gleaming brown, meticulously threaded on a long string of black leather shoelaces.

But old Egghead (his real name was Egget) didn't appreciate either the effort of collecting them or the brilliance of their display. He was furious. And he'd hardly got his breath back from screaming before he'd spotted the string and was flying down the gangway, gown outspread, to seize the end. But this was one prize I wasn't going to give up. With a jerk he succeeded in wrenching the one end away from me, but I held on to the other as fiercely as a rat.

'You can't take these away from me,' I cried, 'I wasn't doing anything with them.'

'How dare you be impertinent to me?' Egghead expostulated.

'Because you're impertinent to me!' I replied.

'I've had my fill of you!' he gasped, his eyes bulging and his eyebrows assuming prominence in his forehead.

'Yes, and I've had my fill of you,' I said, my confidence

mounting since he had failed to act violently to my first rude retort.

He started to pull, but I held on fast. He tried to yank the string out of my hand and I only gripped tighter. Thoughts flashed through my mind as my mental camera stopped on the scene. I wondered what he might do: send me to the Headmaster? threaten me with Detention? or maybe, (I was in a slight frenzy by now) ask me to translate the fight into Latin. I was trying to remember whether the Romans had conker-fights in the arena, and if so, what was the Latin for conker, as we pulled and pulled. I began to imagine myself a Roman, and was determined at all costs that I should win.

Then it happened. The string snapped. It was like the collapse of a tug-of-war team. One minute Egghead was there, the veins throbbing in his huge red face, the next he was gone, catapulting backwards over chairs and desks in a most undignified manner, the broken string waving helplessly in his hands. His foot banged down in front of the desk, then shot right under it. I've never heard such a crack as his head made on that desk. I think the mark's there now if you look carefully. But the conkers . . .

Six feet of them, beautiful, rounded, polished, picked in the full ripeness of Autumn, went rolling in all directions. Down the gangways, beneath the desks, under the blackboard, and out of the room through the French windows. I started to laugh. Then the whole class laughed. They rolled in the aisles till they were hysterical; they had to pick up conkers to keep sane. And when twenty voices were shrieking aloud, and twenty bodies scrabbling furiously over the floor, the Headmaster walked in.

The scene was like an explosion in a marble factory. Some of the boys were lying full length, reaching out under cupboards and bookshelves; others were finding the scattered conkers and then surreptitiously losing them again to prolong the confusion. One boy trod on one and went sailing through the air, his feet whishing from under him. In the background I could vaguely see Egghead being helped to his feet by two over-enthusiastic assistants. They supported him beneath each arm, but his spectacles had been lost in the mêlée, so he only dimly perceived that a new factor had entered the room. He sensed rather than saw the presence of the Headmaster.

Now I had never got on particularly well with old Egghead, but I also knew that neither had the Headmaster been too pleased with his total inability to control even a good-natured class like ours. There had been an incident during the previous term when his Latin class had been taught by one of the boys, complete with cane, gown, and a mortar-board loaned from the Dramatic Society, while he himself had been pleading to be let out of a cupboard. Though he wasn't exactly my best pal, Egghead was at least a fairly decent sort of fellow: after all, he'd played chess for Cambridge, and this impressed me; he had a rather nice wife who sometimes took us home and gave us tea with jam and cream-cakes. One couldn't let this kind of man leave the school without a twinge of conscience, despite the fact that he couldn't teach a word of Latin. (What use was the subject, anyway?)

So as awareness of the impending disaster slowly dawned, I started to think very fast. For Egghead it could be a matter of life or death—his Fate was in the balance.

Finally silence fell. The Head opened his mouth, closed it, opened it again, then as he began to speak I jumped forward.

'Sir!' I gasped, 'the demonstration string broke! Mr Eggh—er—Egget asked me to bring it for a Roman conker fight!' The jubilant class was by now almost seated.

'Sir said that Julius Caesar encouraged his troops in games of skill to while away the time between battles,' I added, beaming brightly. Egghead was standing bravely trying to smile, but holding on firmly to his desk. I think he thought he might go flying again at any minute.

'One of the most popular sports was—er—what did you say the Latin for "chestnut" was, sir?' Egghead cleared his throat horsely, but no sound came out. Then the Head cleared his throat.

'Ah, I see, so this was some kind of—er—demonstration, Mr Egget? Latin through experience, so to speak?' Egghead nodded dumbly. I imagined his tongue sticky-taped to the roof of his mouth. The Head chuckled wanly, then his lips twisted in a strange smile.

'Oh, come, come, Mr Egget, it is obvious you were playing

conkers with the boys—isn't that so, boys?' There was a deathly hush. He smiled sweetly at me. I smiled sweetly back. 'Well, I suppose we're all human, aren't we? No harm in a change from the old grind once in a while, is there?' No-one moved an inch. What was coming next?

'Well, Mr Egget, seeing that you're in such good practice, how about another little contest? You against me, eh? You'd like that, wouldn't you, boys?' And reaching into his pocket he drew out the most gigantic conker I'd ever seen. It was mahogany brown and threaded on an ancient piece of yellow string. It looked as though it had been boiled for thirty years.

Then he fumbled in another pocket and brought out a wad of pound notes. His eyes gleamed wickedly. 'Now, how about a little wager? If I win, Mr Egget, you give me *your* pay packet for the next month. If you win, I surrender *mine*. How's that? That's Roman justice, isn't it, boys?'

There was a murmur of disbelief. Egghead gulped and drew a weary hand across his brow. 'Well, I—er—Mr Headmaster, my wife—'

'Ah, surely you're not going to withdraw from the arena at the critical moment, are you, Mr Egget? Remembering the gladiators, I mean—the net and trident must have been worse, eh? And after all, you *were* giving a demonstration, weren't you?' He grinned maliciously. His massive conker was swaying slightly as he took it in two fingers and raised the string to eye level to test his aim.

'Right, are we ready? Who's going to strike first?' It was Goliath talking to David. But by this time Egghead had one of the champion conkers from my broken string threaded in his hand, and with the class exchanging delighted glances, battle commenced.

Of his own accord the Head took first aim, and let loose with a mighty crack. On impact, Egghead's conker sidled upwards for a moment, rocketed backwards and forwards like a pendulum gone out of its mind, then eventually slowed and resumed a steady equilibrium. It remained unbroken.

'Ha! No easy victory! Well, Mr E, your turn!' The class was now straining forward to get a better view. All eyes were on Egghead as he drew back his gangly arm. The Head's cheeks glowed and his eyes gleamed devilishly under his black brows.

Egghead measured his distance carefully, held his conker precisely between his first and second fingers, then swung. The deadly weapon arched forward and down, only to miss the Head's by a mile, freewheel madly in mid-air, then vanish in the enveloping folds of Egghead's gown. There was a shout of laughter which quickly changed to a fit of coughing. Some of the class were now on their feet.

'So, mine again!' With forehead creased and aim poised, the Head raised his conker a second time and struck viciously. There was another resounding crack, and I closed my eyes, expecting to see the shattered carcass of my precious champion dangling from Egghead's string, but when I looked up both giants were intact. I gasped with relief.

And now, after a further few blows, the battle intensified, as with sweat running down their faces the two struck with ever more deadly aim. The class was now craning excitedly forward, supporting one or other of the opponents and exchanging mouthed bets. The tension was unbearable. Forwards and *crack*! Backwards and *crack*! they went, their muscles standing out in a fury of exertion.

'Come on, sir!' I shouted, cheering on Egghead and hoping the Head wouldn't realize it. Other voices joined in support. I could see Egghead sharing his extra pay packet with us. *Crack*! and *crack*! *Crack*! and *crack*! No quarter was given on either side.

Then suddenly a cry broke from the entire class, now ringed round the two antagonists, as with a final fierce blow a split appeared like a huge erosion on the surface of Egghead's conker. With eyes wild and his breath coming hard, he now stepped back and zoomed his conker forward in a last desperate lunge for victory or defeat. It crashed against the Head's glittering champion with the force of a rock. There was a shattering split that was drowned in a roar, then a sudden silence as the door unexpectedly opened.

A bald head with spectacles balanced on its nose peered around the classroom door. Taking in the scene at a glance, it seemed surprised to see two members of the staff conducting the Latin class, but even more surprised to see a strange object like a half-eaten piece of cheese come floating majestically through the air on what appeared to be a direct collision course with the door. But at the last moment the object seemed to waver in mid-flight, swerve, backfire, and land squarely in the middle of the intruder's nose, sending his spectacles somersaulting through the air onto the wooden platform in front of the board. It was the School Inspector.

'Ah, ha, ho, ah—er—ha, ha, well—now, funny seeing you here, today—of all days—Mr, er—Biggins!' the Head finally managed to stammer out. Then he smiled rather foolishly, in much the same manner as I had smiled at his entry earlier.

'Er, Inspector,' he whispered, 'you—don't—perhaps—happen—to—have—any—*money* on you, do you?'

Manhood *by John Wain*

Swiftly free-wheeling, their breath coming easily, the man and the boy steered their bicycles down the short dip which led them from woodland into open country. Then they looked ahead and saw that the road began to climb.

'Now, Rob,' said Mr Willison, settling his plump haunches firmly on the saddle, 'just up that rise and we'll get off and have a good rest.'

'Can't we rest now?' the boy asked. 'My legs feel all funny. As if they're turning to water.'

'Rest at the top,' said Mr Willison firmly. 'Remember what I told you? The first thing any athlete has to learn is to break the fatigue barrier.'

'I've broken it already. I was feeling tired when we were going along the main road and I—'

'When fatigue sets in, the thing to do is to keep going until it wears off. Then you get your second wind and your second endurance.'

'I've already done that.'

'Up we go,' said Mr Willison, 'and at the top we'll have a good rest.' He panted slightly and stood on his pedals, causing his machine to sway from side to side in a laboured manner. Rob, falling silent, pushed doggedly at his pedals. Slowly, the pair wavered up the straight road to the top. Once there, Mr Willison dismounted with exaggerated steadiness, laid his bicycle carefully on its side, and spread his jacket on the ground before sinking down to rest. Rob slid hastily from the saddle and flung himself full-length on the grass.

'Don't lie there,' said his father. 'You'll catch cold.'

'I'm all right. I'm warm.'

'Come and sit on this. When you're overheated, that's just when you're prone to—'

'I'm all *right*, Dad. I want to lie here. My back aches.'

'Your back needs strengthening, that's why it aches. It's a pity we don't live near a river where you could get some rowing.'

The boy did not answer, and Mr Willison, aware that he was beginning to sound like a nagging, over-anxious parent, allowed himself to be defeated and did not press the suggestion about Rob's coming to sit on his jacket. Instead, he waited a moment and then glanced at his watch.

'Twenty to twelve. We must get going in a minute.'

'*What*? I thought we were going to have a rest.'

'Well, we're having one, aren't we?' said Mr Willison reasonably. 'I've got my breath back, so surely you must have.'

'My back still aches. I want to lie here a bit.'

'Sorry,' said Mr Willison getting up and moving over to his bicycle. 'We've got at least twelve miles to do and lunch is at one.'

'Dad, why did we have to come so far if we've got to get back for one o'clock? I know, let's find a telephone box and ring up Mum and tell her we—'

'Nothing doing. There's no reason why two fit men shouldn't cycle twelve miles in an hour and ten minutes.'

'But we've already done about a million miles.'

'We've done about fourteen, by my estimation,' said Mr Willison stiffly. 'What's the good of going for a bike ride if you don't cover a bit of distance?'

He picked up his bicycle and stood waiting. Rob, with his hand over his eyes, lay motionless on the grass. His legs looked thin and white among the rich grass.

'Come on, Rob.'

The boy showed no sign of having heard. Mr Willison got onto his bicycle and began to ride slowly away. 'Rob,' he called over his shoulder, 'I'm going.'

Rob lay like a sullen corpse by the roadside. He looked horribly like the victim of an accident, unmarked but dead from internal injuries. Mr Willison cycled fifty yards, then a hundred, then turned in a short, irritable circle and came back to where his son lay.

'Rob, is there something the matter or are you just being awkward?'

The boy removed his hand and looked up into his father's face. His eyes were surprisingly mild: there was no fire or rebellion in them.

'I'm tired and my back aches. I can't go on yet.'

'Look, Rob,' said Mr Willison gently, 'I wasn't going to tell you this, because I meant it to be a surprise, but when you get home you'll find a present waiting for you.'

'What kind of present?'

'Something very special I've bought for you. The man's coming this morning to fix it up. That's one reason why I suggested a bike ride this morning. He'll have done it by now.'

'What is it?'

'Aha. It's a surprise. Come on, get on your bike and let's go home and see.'

Rob sat up, then slowly clambered to his feet. 'Isn't there a short cut home?'

'I'm afraid not. It's only twelve miles.'

Rob said nothing.

'And a lot of that's downhill,' Mr Willison added brightly. His own legs were tired and his muscles fluttered unpleasantly. In addition, he suddenly realized he was very thirsty. Rob, still without speaking, picked up his bicycle, and they pedalled away.

'Where is he?' Mrs Willison asked, coming into the garage.

'Gone up to his room,' said Mr Willison. He doubled his fist and gave the punch-ball a thudding blow. 'Seems to have fixed it pretty firmly. You gave him the instructions, I suppose.'

'What's he doing up in his room? It's lunch-time.'

'He said he wanted to rest a bit.'

'I hope you're satisfied,' said Mrs Willison. 'A lad of thirteen, nearly fourteen years of age, just when he should have a really big appetite, and when the lunch is put on the table he's *resting*—'

'Now look, I know what I'm—'

'Lying down in his room, resting, too tired to eat because you've dragged him up hill and down dale on one of your—'

'We did nothing that couldn't be reasonably expected of a boy of his age.'

'How do you know?' Mrs Willison demanded. 'You never did anything of that kind when you were a boy. How do you know what can be reasonably—'

'Now look,' said Mr Willison again. 'When I was a boy, it

was study, study, study all the time, with the fear of unemployment and insecurity in everybody's mind. I was never even given a bicycle. I never boxed, I never rowed, I never did anything to develop my physique. It was just work, work, work, pass this exam, get that certificate. Well, I did it and now I'm qualified and in a secure job. But you know as well as I do that they let me down. Nobody encouraged me to build myself up.'

'Well, what does it matter? You're all right—'

'Grace!' Mr Willison interrupted sharply. 'I am not all right and you know it. I am under average height, my chest is flat and I'm—'

'What nonsense. You're taller than I am and I'm—'

'No son of mine is going to grow up with the same wretched physical heritage that I—'

'No, he'll just have heart disease through over-taxing his strength, because you haven't got the common sense to—'

'His heart is one hundred per cent all right. Not three weeks have gone by since the doctor looked at him.'

'Well, why does he get so over-tired if he's all right? Why is he lying down now instead of coming to the table, a boy of his age?'

A slender shadow blocked part of the dazzling sun in the doorway. Looking up simultaneously, the Willisons greeted their son.

'Lunch ready, Mum? I'm hungry.'

'Ready when you are,' Grace Willison beamed. 'Just wash your hands and come to the table.'

'Look, Rob,' said Mr Willison. 'If you hit with your left hand and then catch it on the rebound with your right, it's excellent ring training.' He dealt the punch-ball two amateurish blows. 'That's what they call a right cross,' he said.

'I think it's fine. I'll have some fun with it,' said Rob. He watched mildly as his father peeled off the padded mittens.

'Here, slip these on,' said Mr Willison. 'They're just training gloves. They harden your fists. Of course, we can get a pair of proper gloves later. But these are specially for use with the ball.'

'Lunch,' called Mrs Willison from the house.

'Take a punch at it,' Mr Willison urged.

'Let's go and eat.'

'Go on. One punch before you go in. I haven't seen you hit it yet.'

Rob took the gloves, put on the right-hand one, and gave the punch-ball one conscientious blow, aiming at the exact centre.

'Now let's go in,' he said.

'Lunch!'

'All right. We're coming . . .'

'Five feet eight, Rob,' said Mr Willison, folding up the wooden ruler. 'You're taller than I am. This is a great landmark.'

'Only just taller.'

'But you're growing all the time. Now all you have to do is to start growing outwards as well as upwards. We'll have you in the middle of that scrum. The heaviest forward in the pack.'

Rob picked up his shirt and began uncertainly poking his arms into the sleeves.

'When do they pick the team?' Mr Willison asked. 'I should have thought they'd have done it by now.'

'They have done it,' said Rob. He bent down to pick up his socks from under a chair.

'They have? And you—'

'I wasn't selected,' said the boy, looking intently at the socks as if trying to detect minute differences in colour and weave.

Mr Willison opened his mouth, closed it again, and stood for a moment looking out of the window. Then he gently laid his hand on his son's shoulder. 'Bad luck,' he said quietly.

'I tried hard,' said Rob quickly.

'I'm sure you did.'

'I played my hardest in the trial games.'

'It's just bad luck,' said Mr Willison. 'It could happen to anybody.'

There was silence as they both continued with their dressing. A faint smell of frying rose into the air, and they could hear Mrs Willison laying the table for breakfast.

'That's it, then, for this season,' said Mr Willison, as if to himself.

'I forgot to tell you, though,' said Rob. 'I was selected for the boxing team.'

'You *were*? I didn't know the school had one.'

'It's new. Just formed. They had some trials for it at the end of last term. I found my punching was better than most people's because I'd been getting plenty of practice with the ball.'

Mr Willison put out a hand and felt Rob's biceps. 'Not bad, not bad at all,' he said critically. 'But if you're going to be a boxer and represent the school, you'll need more power up there. I tell you what. We'll train together.'

'That'll be fun,' said Rob. 'I'm training at school too.'

'What weight do they put you in?'

'It isn't weight, it's age. Under fifteen. Then when you get over fifteen you get classified into weights.'

'Well,' said Mr Willison, tying his tie, 'you'll be in a good position for the under-fifteens. You've got six months to play with. And there's no reason why you shouldn't steadily put muscle on all the time. I suppose you'll be entered as a team, for tournaments and things?'

'Yes. There's a big one at the end of next term. I'll be in that.'

Confident, joking, they went down to breakfast. 'Two eggs for Rob, Mum,' said Mr Willison. 'He's in training. He's going to be a heavyweight.'

'A heavyweight what?' Mrs Willison asked, teapot in hand.

'Boxer,' Rob smiled.

Grace Willison put down the teapot, her lips compressed, and looked from one to the other. '*Boxing*?' she repeated.

'Boxing,' Mr Willison replied calmly.

'Over my dead body,' said Mrs Willison. 'That's one sport I'm definite that he's never going in for.'

'Too late. They've picked him for the under-fifteens. He's had trials and everything.'

'Is this true, Rob?' she demanded.

'Yes,' said the boy, eating rapidly.

'Well, you can just tell them you're dropping it. Baroness Summerskill—'

'To hell with Baroness Summerskill!' her husband shouted. 'The first time he gets a chance to do something, the first time he gets picked for a team and given a chance to show what he's made of, and you have to bring up Baroness Summerskill.'

'But it injures their brains! All those blows on the front of the skull. I've read about it—'

'Injures their brains!' Mr Willison snorted. 'Has it injured Ingemar Johansson's brain? Why, he's one of the acutest business men in the world!'

'Rob,' said Mrs Willison steadily, 'when you get to school, go and see the sports master and tell him you're giving up boxing.'

'There isn't a sports master. All the masters do bits of it at different times.'

'There must be one who's in charge of boxing. All you have to do is tell him—'

'Are you ready, Rob?' said Mr Willison. 'You'll be late for school if you don't go.'

'I'm in plenty of time, Dad. I haven't finished my breakfast.'

'Never mind, push along, old son. You've had your egg and bacon, that's what matters. I want to talk to your mother.'

Cramming a piece of dry toast in his mouth, the boy picked up his satchel and wandered from the room. Husband and wife sat back, glaring hot-eyed at each other.

The quarrel began, and continued for many days. In the end it was decided that Rob should continue boxing until he had represented the school at the tournament in March of the following year, and should then give it up.

'Ninety-six, ninety-seven, ninety-eight, ninety-nine, a hundred,' Mr Willison counted. 'Right, that's it. Now go and take your shower and get into bed.'

'I don't feel tired, honestly,' Rob protested.

'Who's manager here, you or me?' Mr Willison asked bluffly. 'I'm in charge of training and you can't say my methods don't work. Fifteen solid weeks and you start questioning my decisions on the very night of the fight?'

'It just seems silly to go to bed when I'm not—'

'My dear Rob, please trust me. No boxer ever went into a big fight without spending an hour or two in bed, resting, just before going to his dressing-room.'

'All right, but I bet none of the others are bothering to do all this.'

'That's exactly why you're going to be better than the

others. Now go and get your shower before you catch cold. Leave the skipping-rope, I'll put it away.'

After Rob had gone, Mr Willison folded the skipping-rope into a neat ball and packed it away in the case that contained the boy's gloves, silk dressing-gown, lace-up boxing boots, and trunks with the school badge sewn into the correct position on the right leg. There would be no harm in a little skipping, to limber up and conquer his nervousness while waiting to go on. Humming, he snapped down the catches of the small leather case and went into the house.

Mrs Willison did not lift her eyes from the television set as he entered. 'All ready now, Mother,' said Mr Willison. 'He's going to rest in bed now, and go along at about six o'clock. I'll go with him and wait till the doors open to be sure of a ringside seat.' He sat down on the sofa beside his wife, and tried to put his arm round her. 'Come on, love,' he said coaxingly. 'Don't spoil my big night.'

She turned to him and he was startled to see her eyes brimming with angry tears. 'What about my big night?' she asked, her voice harsh. 'Fourteen years ago, remember? When he came into the world.'

'Well, what about it?' Mr Willison parried, uneasily aware that the television set was quacking and signalling on the fringe of his attention, turning the scene from clumsy tragedy into a clumsier farce.

'Why didn't you tell me then?' she sobbed. 'Why did you let me have a son if all you were interested in was having him punched to death by a lot of rough bullet-headed louts who—'

'Take a grip on yourself, Grace. A punch on the nose won't hurt him.'

'You're an unnatural father,' she keened. 'I don't know how you can bear to send him into that ring to be beaten and thumped—Oh, why can't you stop him now? Keep him at home? There's no *law* that compels us to—'

'That's where you're wrong, Grace,' said Mr Willison sternly. 'There is a law. The unalterable law of nature that says that young males of the species indulge in manly trials of strength. Think of all the other lads who are going into the ring tonight. D'you think their mothers are sitting about crying and kicking up a fuss? No—they're proud to have strong, masculine sons who can stand up in the ring and take a few punches.'

'Go away, please,' said Mrs Willison, sinking back with closed eyes. 'Just go right away and don't come near me until it's all over.'

'Grace!'

'Please. Please leave me alone. I can't bear to look at you and I can't bear to hear you.'

'You're hysterical,' said Mr Willison bitterly. Rising, he went out into the hall and called up the stairs. 'Are you in bed, Rob?'

There was a slight pause and then Rob's voice called faintly, 'Could you come up, Dad?'

'Come up? Why? Is something the matter?'

'Could you come up?'

Mr Willison ran up the stairs. 'What is it?' he panted. 'D'you want something?'

'I think I've got appendicitis,' said Rob. He lay squinting among the pillows, his face suddenly narrow and crafty.

'I don't believe you,' said Mr Willison shortly. 'I've supervised your training for fifteen weeks and I know you're as fit as a fiddle. You can't possibly have anything wrong with you.'

'I've got a terrible pain in my side,' said Rob. 'Low down on the right-hand side. That's where appendicitis comes, isn't it?'

Mr Willison sat down on the bed. 'Listen, Rob,' he said. 'Don't do this to me. All I'm asking you to do is to go into the ring and have one bout. You've been picked for the school team and everyone's depending on you.'

'I'll die if you don't get the doctor,' Rob suddenly hissed. 'Mum!' he shouted.

Mrs Willison came bounding up the stairs. 'What is it, my pet?'

'My stomach hurts. Low down on the right-hand side.'

'Appendicitis!' She whirled to face Mr Willison. 'That's what comes of your foolishness!'

'I don't believe it,' said Mr Willison. He went out of the bedroom and down the stairs. The television was still jabbering in the living-room, and for fifteen minutes Mr Willison forced himself to sit staring at the strident puppets, glistening in metallic light, as they enacted their Lilliputian rituals. Then he went up to the bedroom again. Mrs Willison was bathing Rob's forehead.

'His temperature's normal,' she said.

'Of course his temperature's normal,' said Mr Willison. 'He doesn't want to fight, that's all.'

'Fetch the doctor,' said a voice from under the cold flannel that swathed Rob's face.

'We will, pet, if you don't get better very soon,' said Mrs Willison, darting a murderous glance at her husband.

Mr Willison slowly went downstairs. For a moment he stood looking at the telephone, then picked it up and dialled the number of the grammar school. No-one answered. He replaced the receiver, went to the foot of the stairs and called, 'What's the name of the master in charge of this tournament?'

'I don't know,' Rob called weakly.

'You told me you'd been training with Mr Granger,' Mr Willison called. 'Would he know anything about it?'

Rob did not answer, so Mr Willison looked up all the Grangers in the telephone book. There were four in the town, but only one was MA. 'That's him,' said Mr Willison. With lead in his heart and ice on his fingers he dialled the number.

Mrs Granger fetched Mr Granger. Yes, he taught at the school. He was the right man. What could he do for Mr Willison?

'It's about tonight's boxing tournament.'

'Sorry, what? The line's bad.'

'Tonight's boxing tournament.'

'Have you got the right person?'

'You teach my son, Rob—we've just agreed on that. Well, it's about the boxing tournament he's supposed to be taking part in tonight.'

'Where?'

'Where? At the school, of course. He's representing the under-fifteens.'

There was a pause. 'I'm not quite sure what mistake you're making, Mr Willison, but I think you've got hold of the wrong end of at least one stick.' A hearty, defensive laugh. 'If Rob belongs to a boxing club it's certainly news to me, but in any case it can't be anything to do with the school. We don't go in for boxing.'

'Don't go in for it?'

'We don't offer it. It's not in our curriculum.'

'Oh,' said Mr Willison. 'Oh. Thank you. I must have—well, thank you.'

'Not at all. I'm glad to answer any queries. Everything's all right, I trust?'

'Oh, yes,' said Mr Willison, 'yes, thanks. Everything's all right.'

He put down the telephone, hesitated, then turned and began slowly to climb the stairs.

Lady of the Ice *by Sheila Markowitz*

Maria's mother used to tell her that she had been born with skates on her feet. There was an old Russian legend that spoke of a Lady of the Ice and Snow. One summer she had been unfaithful to her lover and as a result he would only return to her in winter when the trees were garbed with snow and the lakes frozen hard with ice. They would then skate together for a season before the Caucasian wind would bring the Spring, and she would be left to mourn until his return.

Her mother often called Maria the 'Lady of the Ice'. She had skated as long as she could remember. While still a young girl she had mastered the complex figure-eights, reverse turns, spins and glides. In her teens she could perform pirouettes and arabesques with grace, and later, with her partner, could match the finest dancers, executing elaborate movements with ease.

The year that her mother died, Maria became attached to a touring ballet company. And it was here that she met Pierre. In his arms she felt as secure as any partner could be. He taught her to relax in the swing when she would float away from his body at arm's length; he showed her how to breathe naturally as she sped inches from the ground in a breathtaking whirl. One moment she would be in the air, the next thrown back against the floor, another floating with arms outstretched, horizontal to his waist, but always held firm and sure like an aerial figurine.

Her exquisite dancing won acclaim and soon she became a star. She drew capacity audiences and rave notices from the press. As a pair she and Pierre were praised wherever they went.

About this time a boy called Andrei had been engaged to design the company's costumes. Not being a skater himself, he would sit watching from the rink side as Maria and Pierre perfected their movements. He grew to love Maria's slender body that seemed to manipulate the very air itself. Gradually he fell in love with her.

Sheila Markowitz

One day in her dressing-room Maria found a parcel with her name on it. On opening it she drew forth the most scintillating dress she had ever seen: a scarlet bodice ringed with shimmering brilliants. There was no indication as to the sender, but it didn't take long to discover his identity. She had begun to notice her silent admirer sitting day after day by the rink side, spending every free moment watching her. Flattered by Andrei's affections, she had secretly begun to reciprocate his love, though no word had actually passed between them.

On the day following the arrival of the gift, she approached him in between practice sessions.

'You shouldn't have been so kind,' she remonstrated, delighted at the pleasure it gave him to receive her thanks.

They met frequently afterwards, and often referred to the dress as his gift of love. He lavished every attention on her, and she responded warmly as it was her nature to do. Only occasionally would he appear lonely and depressed as he sat without her; at other times he would watch, ravished by her dancing, at the rink side.

Some months later they were married. As part of her wedding gift he designed a dazzling dress with cloak to match, and on the label wrote: 'To my Lady of the Ice'.

For a time they were happy, finding joy in each other's nearness. His love was spontaneous, possessive and warm. But a few months after their marriage, when he had spent a day watching her prepare for a gala performance, he suggested that perhaps she should take a rest from dancing for a while. Oh no, she exclaimed, dancing was her life: how could she ever tire of it? He let the matter rest, but a few weeks later, after a particularly successful performance, he renewed his request. Wouldn't she take a break from her work and enjoy a sightseeing tour with him? Yes, she replied, she would love a tour, but of course they must wait until the season ended. Then seeing his face twisted in annoyance, she cried, 'Why, Andrei, whatever is the matter? You used to delight in seeing me dance!'

'I like you to dance, but I would prefer it to be with someone else,' he answered abruptly.

'But Pierre is a wonderful dancer!' she exclaimed, and then, seeing his expression, realized her mistake. He was insanely jealous. Since first he had seen her dance so serenely, he had had to watch her for hours and days in the arms of another man.

'But I don't love Pierre!' she cried. 'Andrei, you know I think only of you!' Her protestations were in vain. Even mention of her partner's name repulsed him and would induce a fit of angry depression. He left the room without a word.

From then on matters became worse. Maria felt bound to her partner and obliged to finish the season with him, even if she had to relinquish him later, which in her heart she didn't wish to do. Her love for her husband, which was deep and real, began to vie with her love for her work. Her performances, once so faultless, began to deteriorate. The crowds sensed her uncertainty; and above all her tension began to affect Pierre.

'Maria, what has come over you?' he asked one night after a disturbing performance during which she made a movement that almost led to a fall. 'You seem so nervous and ill at ease.'

'I'm sorry, I can't seem to concentrate,' she cried. 'I think I need a rest,' and she hurried home, sick with anxiety. Andrei was out. He had stopped coming to watch her, and she knew that they were in danger of drifting apart. When he eventually returned he was sullen and uncommunicative. He had been drinking heavily.

The care she offered him was to no avail. Her despair grew and her performance worsened. One day the strain became too great: she was listless and Pierre was angry.

'How can I dance with you as you are, Maria?' he exclaimed. 'I must know what is wrong with you.' Distraught, she told him. He listened gravely. 'But Maria,' he said, 'you and I are only dancing partners. I admire you, but as an artist.' Yet inwardly he knew that he was not speaking the truth, and Maria realized it even as he spoke. He loved her as a woman as well as for her professional excellence. And though he tried to soothe her, he had no solution to offer, nor did he desire to lose her.

One night before a double performance at the Moscow Arts Theatre she felt particularly tired and brittle, and had first pleaded, then argued with her husband. Why should she give up the partner who had brought her success? How could

Andrei be so heartless as to threaten her career? His cancerous jealousy was destroying their happiness.

When she returned home after the performance it was late, but he was not to be found. After waiting an hour she grew anxious and decided to drive out in the car to meet him. The night was dark and starless, but two miles from their home she found him wandering by the roadside, hopelessly drunk. When she opened the car door and called to him, he swore at her, then lurched in and grabbed hold of the wheel, pushing her aside.

'No, Andrei, no!' she cried, as he banged the door and started to drive.

'Who the hell are you talking to?' he said thickly, 'can't I drive my own car?' Overcome with fear and distress she tried to reason with him, but he engaged gear and accelerated for home. The car began to swerve from one side of the road to the other, until as they approached a small bridge she could bear it no longer and put her hand on the wheel to save them from disaster. With a wrench he spun it away and to her terror-stricken cry the car left the road, vaulted over the bridge, and grounded in a nearby field.

Maria spent a month convalescing. She had come out of the accident unscathed except for a broken arm and a leg which had been trapped. The arm would soon heal, but the leg was badly crushed. On crutches she managed to move around: slowly at first, then more smoothly, but with a pronounced limp. Of her husband there had been no word.

It was a year and a half before her leg was fully healed. Many sympathizers had come to visit her, and she had received countless letters of condolence and offers of help. She welcomed them all gladly, but when they spoke of her dancing loss, she felt the deeper loss of the husband she had once treasured and loved. He had disappeared, seemingly without trace.

In the second year she was able to skate once again. Pierre was dancing as brilliantly as ever, but with a new partner, and though he treated her kindly, she sensed a remoteness.

When first she ventured onto the ice again she was tentative and afraid, but gradually she became accustomed to it, regained her poise, and apart from an occasional twinge of pain, felt completely recovered.

To fill up her time she joined a new ballet company in the suburbs and performed a minor act with something of her former grace, but none of the ease which had won her acclaim. She practised relentlessly, and always in between dances would glance at the stands to see if one particular man was watching her. One day she thought she caught a glimpse of him disappearing through a door; at another performance she was certain there had been someone resembling him in the background; but the lights dazzled her, and when she went back to look for him he was gone.

Then, after a period of loneliness, she saw him. He was wearing a heavy overcoat and beard, and stood half-concealed behind a pillar at an evening performance. Determined not to let him escape, she pretended not to see him, then after her act, changed quickly and ran round to the entrance to speak to him as he came out. There was no bitterness in her intentions. She felt regretful of her own impulsiveness and wanted only to forgive him, and now that his rival was gone, to begin life anew.

But even as she stood there in the shadows she knew that he had been too quick for her. Already he was on the opposite side of the street and turning down an alleyway. In panic she called to him, but her words were muffled by the snow, and in a moment he was out of sight. She began to run desperately now, at first calling, then saving her breath for the effort of running, but she couldn't match his speed. He went on for several minutes, always ahead, sometimes hidden, sometimes just in sight. They had left the theatre far behind and were crossing a waste patch of ground. She was in the distance when he approached a grimy block of flats. She saw him enter and struggled on frantically, glimpsing him for a moment behind thin curtains as a light flickered on and off. By the time she reached it, the building was in darkness.

Summoning all her strength, she rushed up a single flight of stairs and knocked on the door, but there was no reply. It opened at a touch. There were signs of recent habitation, but no sign of him. She looked in the kitchen, but there were only a few unwashed dishes and beer cans piled in the corner. From the window she fancied she heard a sound in the distance, but when she looked she could see nothing.

Crushed and desperate, she trudged back to the theatre, then returned to her own home only to find that someone had been there. The door had been opened and a package lay in the middle of the table. Trembling, she picked it up and tore off the flimsy wrapper. Inside was a skater's gown of radiant black and emerald velvet and from it dangled a scrawled label with the words: 'To the Lady of the Ice'.

She never saw him again. But as she skated alone on the glittering ice under myriad lights her eyes would sometimes blur, and in that moment she would see a thousand faces following her every movement, and know that every one of them was Andrei: watching, watching, watching.

Little Old Lady from Cricket Creek

by Len Gray

Art Bowen and I were trying to analyse performance evaluations when Penny Thorpe, my secretary, walked into the office.

'Yeah, Penny. What's up?'

'Mr Cummings, there's a woman out in the lobby. She's applying for the filing clerk's job.' Penny walked over and laid the application form on my desk.

'Good, good. I only hope she's not one of those high-school drop-outs we've been getting.' I stopped, staring at the form. 'Age sixty-five! What the hell are we running around here? A playground for Whistler's mother?'

Art put his Roman nose in it. 'Now, Ralph, let's take it easy. Maybe the old gal's a good worker. We can't kick 'em out of the building just because they've been around a few years. How's the application?'

Good old Art. Always the peacemaker.

'Well,' I said doubtfully, 'it says her name is Mabel Jumpstone. That's right. Jumpstone. Good experience. Seems qualified. You game for an interview?'

'Sure. Why not? Let's do one together.'

This is against the company policy of Great Riveroak Insurance Company. All personnel interviewers are to conduct separate interviews and make individual decisions—at least that's what we're supposed to do. Usually we double up and save time.

Penny remained standing in front of my desk, tapping her pencil. 'Well?' she asked haughtily, which sums up her disposition perfectly.

'OK, Penny. Send Mrs Jumpstone in.'

Mrs Jumpstone came shuffling into the office, smiling and nodding her head like an old grey mare. Her black outfit looked like pre-World War I. She had on a purple hat with pink plastic flowers round the brim.

She sat down and said, 'Hello there!' Her voice was almost a bellow.

I looked at Art, who was leaning forward in his chair, his mouth open, his eyes round.

'Er . . . Mrs Jumpstone,' I began.

'Mabel. Please.'

'OK, Mabel. This is Mr Bowen, my associate.' I waved a hand at Art, who mumbled something inappropriate. 'This is a very interesting application, Mabel. It says here you were born in Cricket Creek, California.'

'That's right, young man. Home of John and Mary Jackson.'

She smiled at me, proud of the information.

Art bent over, scratching his wrist. 'John and Mary Jackson?'

'Oh, yes,' she replied, 'the gladiolus-growers.'

He tried to smile. I'll give him credit. 'The—the—oh, yes, of course. It must have slipped my mind. Let me see that application, Ralph.' He grabbed it from the desk and took a few minutes to study it thoroughly.

Mabel and I sat and watched each other. Every once in a while she'd wink. I tried looking at the ceiling.

Art glanced up and snapped, 'You worked at Upstate California Insurance for ten years. Why did you quit?' Sharp-thinking Art. He made a career of trying to catch people off guard. I'd never seen him do it yet.

Mabel shrugged her tiny shoulders. 'Young man, have you ever lived up North? It's another world. Cold and foggy. I just had to leave. I told Harry—that's my husband, who passed away recently, God rest his soul—that we had to come down here. Mr Bowen, you wouldn't believe how much I enjoy the sun. Of course, you've never been in Cricket Creek,' she added, which was true, of course. I doubted very much if Art had even heard of Cricket Creek.

Art looked as if he wanted to hide. Mabel smiled brightly at him, nodding her head pleasantly.

'Mabel,' I said, 'the job we have open entails keeping our personnel files up to date. Quite a bit of work, you know, in an office this size.'

'Really?'

'Really. It even requires a bit of typing. You *can* type?'

'Oh, heavens, yes. Would you like me to take a test?'

'Er . . . yes, that might be a good idea. Let's go and find a typewriter. Coming, Art?'

He grinned. 'Wouldn't miss it for the world.'

We walked out of the office. Art whispered in my ear, 'About ten words a minute would be my guess.'

It turned out to be more like ninety: I handed Mabel one of our surveys on employee retention and told her to have a go at it. She handled the typewriter like a machine-gun. The carriage kept clicking back and forth so fast that Art almost got a sore neck watching the keys fly.

Our applicant handed me three pages. I couldn't find a single error. Art looked over each page as if he were examining the paper for fingerprints. He finally gave up, shaking his head.

Mabel went back to my office. Art and I walked over to a corner, Art holding the typed sheets.

'Well, what do you think?' he asked.

'She's the best typist in the building. Definitely. Without a doubt.'

She's different. But you're right. Check her references.'

'And if they're OK?'

He shrugged. 'Let's hire ourselves a little old lady from Cricket Creek.'

Art poked his head in my door the next day. 'What about our typewriter whiz?'

'I just called her to offer her the job. Application checked out perfectly.'

He laughed. 'I bet she raises a few eyebrows.'

In fact, within two months Mabel Jumpstone was the most popular employee in the building. Whenever someone had a birthday she brought in a cake and served it during the afternoon break. And people with problems started coming to her. She arrived early each morning and stayed late. She never missed a day off work. Not one.

Six months after we hired her, Art walked slowly into my office. His eyes were glassy and his mouth was slack. He slumped down heavily in a chair.

'What's the matter with you?' I asked.

'The cash mail,' he groaned.

We receive quite a lot of cash from our customers. Once a week, on Friday, we take it to the bank. It was Friday.

'What about the cash mail, Art? Come on, what's the matter?'

He looked at me, blinking. 'Harvey was taking it to the bank.

He called ten minutes ago. He was robbed. Conked. Knocked out. And guess who did it?'

'Who?'

'Mabel. Mabel Jumpstone. Our little old lady.'

'You're kidding. You've got to be *kidding*, Art.'

He shook his head. 'Harvey said she wanted a lift to the bank. After they got going, she took a pistol out of her handbag and told him to pull over. Harvey said it looked like a cannon. The gun, I mean. He's just woken up. The money and Harvey's car are gone. So's Mabel.'

I stared at him. 'I can't believe it!'

'It's true. Every word. What are we going to do?'

I snapped my fingers. 'The application! Come on.'

We ran to the filing cabinets and opened the one labelled 'Employees'. The application was gone, of course. There was a single sheet inside the manila folder. It was typed very neatly. '*I resign. Sincerely yours, Mabel.*' The name had been typed, too. There was no handwritten signature. Mabel had never written anything. She always insisted on everything being typed.

Art stared at me. 'Do you remember anything on the application? Anything? The references?' He was pleading.

'For Pete's sake, Art, it was six months ago!' I paused for a moment. 'I can remember *one* thing. Just one.'

'What?'

'She came from Cricket Creek. I wonder if there *is* a Cricket Creek?'

We checked.

There wasn't.

I finally got home to my two-bedroom bachelor apartment late that evening. The police had been sympathetic. Real nice to us. They didn't even laugh when we told them they were after a little old lady of sixty-five. They asked for a photograph or a sample of handwriting.

We didn't have either.

I opened a can of beer and then walked into one of the bedrooms.

Mabel was sitting on the bed, neatly counting $78,000 into two separate piles.

I looked at her, smiled, and said, 'Hi, Mom.'

The Secret Life of Walter Mitty

by James Thurber

'We're going through!' The Commander's voice was like thin ice breaking. He wore his full-dress uniform, with the heavily braided white cap pulled down rakishly over one cold grey eye. 'We can't make it, sir. It's spoiling for a hurricane, if you ask me.' 'I'm not asking you, Lieutenant Berg,' said the Commander. 'Throw on the power lights! Rev her up to 8500! We're going through!' The pounding of the cylinders increased: ta-pocketa-pocketa-pocketa-*pocketa-pocketa*. The Commander stared at the ice forming on the pilot window. He walked over and twisted a row of complicated dials. 'Switch on No 8 auxiliary!' he shouted. 'Switch on No 8 auxiliary!' repeated Lieutenant Berg. 'Full strength in No 3 turret!' shouted the Commander. 'Full strength in No 3 turret!' The crew, bending to their various tasks in the huge, hurtling eight-engined Navy hydroplane, looked at each other and grinned. 'The Old Man'll get us through,' they said to one another. 'The Old Man ain't afraid of Hell!' . . .

'Not so fast! You're driving too fast!' said Mrs Mitty. 'What are you driving so fast for?'

'Hmm?' said Walter Mitty. He looked at his wife in the seat beside him with shocked astonishment. She seemed grossly unfamiliar, like a strange woman who had yelled at him in a crowd. 'You were up to fifty-five,' she said. 'You know I don't like to go more than forty. You were up to fifty-five.' Walter Mitty drove on towards Waterbury in silence, the roaring of the SN202 through the worst storm in twenty years of Navy flying fading in the remote, intimate airways of his mind. 'You're tensed up again,' said Mrs Mitty. 'It's one of your days. I wish you'd let Dr Renshaw look you over.'

Walter Mitty stopped the car in front of the building where his wife went to have her hair done. 'Remember to get those overshoes while I'm having my hair done,' she said. 'I don't need overshoes,' said Mitty. She put her mirror back into her bag. 'We've been through all that,' she said, getting out of the car. 'You're not a young man any longer.' He raced the engine a little. 'Why don't you wear your gloves? Have you lost your gloves?' Walter Mitty reached in a pocket and brought out the gloves. He put them on, but after she had turned and gone into the building and he had driven on to a red light, he took them off again. 'Pick it up, brother!' snapped a cop as the lights changed, and Mitty hastily pulled on his gloves and lurched ahead. He drove round the streets aimlessly for a time, and then he drove past the hospital on his way back to the parking lot.

. . . 'It's the millionaire banker, Wellington McMillan,' said the pretty nurse. 'Yes?' said Walter Mitty, removing his gloves slowly. 'Who has the case?' 'Dr Renshaw and Dr Benbow, but there are two specialists here, Dr Remington from New York and Mr Pritchard-Mitford from London. He flew over.' A door opened down a long, cool corridor and Dr Renshaw came out. He looked distraught and haggard. 'Hello, Mitty,' he said. 'We're having the devil's own time with McMillan, the millionaire banker and close personal friend of Roosevelt. Obstreosis of the ductal tract. Tertiary. Wish you'd take a look at him.' 'Glad to,' said Mitty.

In the operating room there were whispered introductions: 'Dr Remington, Dr Mitty, Mr Pritchard-Mitford, Dr Mitty.' 'I've read your book on streptothricosis,' said Pritchard-Mitford, shaking hands. 'A brilliant performance, sir.' 'Thank you,' said Walter Mitty. 'Didn't know you were in the States, Mitty,' grumbled Remington. 'Coals to Newcastle, bringing Mitford and me up here for a tertiary.' 'You are very kind,' said Mitty. A huge, complicated machine, connected to the operating table with many tubes and wires, began at this moment to go pocketa-pocketa-pocketa. 'The new anaesthetizer is giving way!' shouted an intern. 'There is no-one in the East who knows how to fix it!' 'Quiet man!' said Mitty, in a low cool voice. He sprang to the machine, which was now going pocketa-pocketa-queep-pocketa-queep. He began fingering delicately a row of glistening dials. 'Give me a fountain pen!' he snapped. Someone handed him a fountain pen. He pulled a faulty piston out of the machine and inserted the pen in its place. 'That will hold for ten minutes,' he said. 'Get on with the operation.' A nurse hurried over and whispered to Renshaw, and Mitty saw the man turn pale. 'Coreopsis has set in,' said Renshaw nervously. 'If you would take over, Mitty?' Mitty looked at him and at the craven figure of Benbow, who drank, and at the grave uncertain faces of the two great specialists. 'If you wish,' he said. They slipped a white gown on him; he adjusted a mask and drew on thin gloves; nurses handed him shining . . .

'Back it up, Mac! Look out for that Buick!' Walter Mitty jammed on the brakes. 'Wrong lane, Mac,' said the parking-lot attendant, looking at Mitty closely. 'Gee. Yeh,' muttered Mitty. He began cautiously to back out of the lane marked 'Exit Only'. 'Leave her sit there,' said the attendant. 'I'll put her away.' Mitty got out of the car. 'Hey, better leave the key.' 'Oh,' said Mitty, handing the man the ignition key. The attendant vaulted into the car, backed it up with insolent skill, and put it where it belonged.

They're so damned cocky, thought Walter Mitty, walking along Main Street: they think they know everything. Once he had tried to take his chains off outside New Milford, and he had got them wound round the axles. A man had had to come out in a wrecking-car and unwind them, a young, grinning garageman. Since then Mrs Mitty always made him drive to a garage to have the chains taken off. The next time, he thought, I'll wear my right arm in a sling; they won't grin at me then. I'll have my right arm in a sling and they'll see I couldn't possibly take the chains off myself. He kicked at the slush on the sidewalk. 'Overshoes,' he said to himself, and he began looking for a shoe store.

When he came out into the street again with the overshoes in a box under his arm, Walter Mitty began to wonder what the other thing was his wife had told him to get. She had told him twice, before they set out from their house for Waterbury. In a way he hated these weekly trips to town—he was always getting something wrong. Kleenex, he thought, Squibb's, razor blades? No. Toothpaste, toothbrush, bicarbonate, carborundum, initiative and referendum? He gave it up. But she would remember it. 'Where's the what's-its-name?' she would ask. 'Don't tell me you forgot the what's-its-name.' A newsboy went by shouting something about the Waterbury trial.

. . . 'Perhaps this will refresh your memory.' The District Attorney suddenly thrust a heavy automatic at the quiet figure on the witness stand. 'Have you ever seen this before?' Walter Mitty took the gun and examined it expertly. 'This is my Webley-Vickers 50.80,' he said calmly. An excited buzz ran around the courtroom. The judge rapped for order. 'You are a crack shot with any sort of firearms, I believe?' said the District Attorney insinuatingly. 'Objection!' shouted Mitty's attorney. 'We have shown that the defendant could not have fired the shot. We have shown that he wore his right arm in a sling on the night of the fourteenth of July.' Walter Mitty raised his hand briefly and the bickering attorneys were stilled. 'With any known make of gun,' he said evenly, 'I could have killed Gregory Fitzhurst at three hundred feet *with my left hand.*' Pandemonium broke loose in the courtroom. A woman's scream rose above the bedlam and suddenly a lovely, dark-haired girl was in Walter Mitty's arms. The District Attorney struck at her savagely. Without rising from his chair, Mitty let the man have it on the point of the chin. 'You miserable cur!' . . .

'Puppy biscuit,' said Walter Mitty. He stopped walking and the buildings of Waterbury rose up out of the misty courtroom and surrounded him again. A woman who was passing laughed. 'He said "Puppy biscuit",' she said to her companion. 'That man said "Puppy biscuit" to himself.' Walter Mitty hurried on. He went into an A & P, not the first one he came to but a smaller one farther up the street. 'I want some biscuit for small, young dogs,' he said to the clerk. 'Any special brand, sir?' The greatest pistol shot in the world thought a moment. 'It says "Puppies Bark for It" on the box,' said Walter Mitty.

His wife would be through at the hairdresser's in fifteen minutes, Mitty saw in looking at his watch, unless they had trouble drying it; sometimes they had trouble drying it. She didn't like to get to the hotel first: she would want him to be there waiting for her as usual. He found a big leather chair in the lobby facing a window, and he put the overshoes and the puppy biscuit on the floor beside it. He picked up an old copy of *Liberty* and sank down into the chair. 'Can Germany Conquer the World Through the Air?' Walter Mitty looked at the pictures of bombing planes and of ruined streets.

. . . 'The cannonading has got the wind up in young Raleigh, sir,' said the sergeant. Captain Mitty looked up at him through tousled hair. 'Get him to bed,' he said wearily. 'With the others. I'll fly alone.' 'But you can't sir,' said the sergeant anxiously. 'It takes two men to handle that bomber and the Archies are pounding hell out of the air. Von Richtman's circus is between here and Saulier.' 'Somebody's got to get that ammunition dump,' said Mitty. 'I'm going over. Spot of brandy?' He poured a drink for the sergeant and one for himself. War thundered and whined around the dugout and battered at the door. There was a rend of wood, and splinters flew through the room. 'A bit of a near thing,' said Captain Mitty carelessly. 'The box barrage is closing in,' said the sergeant. 'We only live once, Sergeant,' said Mitty, with his faint, fleeting smile. 'Or do we?' He poured another brandy and tossed it off. 'I never see a man could hold his brandy like you, sir,' said the sergeant. 'Begging your pardon, sir.' Captain Mitty stood up and strapped on his huge Webley-Vickers automatic. 'It's forty kilometres through hell, sir,' said the sergeant. Mitty finished one last brandy. 'After all,' he said softly, 'what isn't?' The pounding of the cannon increased: there was the rat-tat-tatting of machine-guns, and from somewhere came the menacing pocketa-pocketa-pocketa of the new flamethrowers. Walter Mitty walked to the door of the dugout humming 'Auprès de Ma Blonde'. He turned and waved to the sergeant. 'Cheerio!' he said . . .

Something struck his shoulder. 'I've been looking all over this hotel for you,' said Mrs Mitty. 'Why do you have to hide in this old chair? How do you expect me to find you?' 'Things close in,' said Walter Mitty vaguely. 'What?' Mrs Mitty said. 'Did you get the what's-its-name? The puppy biscuit? What's in that box?' 'Overshoes,' said Mitty. 'Couldn't you have put them on in the store?' 'I was thinking,' said Walter Mitty. 'Does it ever occur to you that I am sometimes thinking?' She looked at him. 'I'm going to take your temperature when I get you home,' she said.

They went out through the revolving doors that made a faintly derisive whistling sound when you pushed them. It was two blocks to the parking lot. At the drugstore on the corner she said, 'Wait here for me. I forgot something. I won't be a minute.' She was more than a minute. Walter Mitty lit a cigarette. It began to rain, rain with sleet in it. He stood up against the wall of the drugstore, smoking . . . He put his shoulders back and his heels together. 'To hell with the handkerchief,' said Walter Mitty scornfully. He took one last drag on his cigarette and snapped it away. Then, with that faint, fleeting smile playing about his lips, he faced the firing squad: erect and motionless, proud and disdainful, Walter Mitty the Undefeated, inscrutable to the last.

The Ruum *by Arthur Porges*

The cruiser *Ilkor* had just gone into her interstellar overdrive beyond the orbit of Pluto when a worried officer reported to the Commander.

'Excellency,' he said uneasily. 'I regret to inform you that because of a technician's carelessness a Type H-9 Ruum has been left behind on the third planet, together with anything it may have collected.'

The Commander's triangular eyes hooded momentarily, but when he spoke his voice was level.

'How was the ruum set?'

'For a maximum radius of 30 miles, and 160 pounds plus or minus 15.'

There was silence for several seconds, then the Commander said: 'We cannot reverse course now. In a few weeks we'll be returning, and can pick up the ruum then. I do not care to have one of these costly, self-energizing models charged against my ship. You will see,' he ordered coldly, 'that the individual responsible is severely punished.'

But at the end of its run, in the neighbourhood of Rigel, the cruiser met a flat, ring-shaped raider; and when the inevitable fire-fight was over, both ships, semi-molten, radioactive, and laden with dead, were starting a billion-year orbit around the star.

And on the earth, it was the age of reptiles.

When the two men had unloaded the last of the supplies, Jim Irwin watched his partner climb into the little seaplane. He waved at Walt.

'Don't forget to mail that letter to my wife,' Jim shouted.

'The minute I land,' Walt Leonard called back, starting to rev the engine. 'And you find us some uranium—a strike is just what Cele needs. A fortune for your son and her, hey?' His white teeth flashed in a grin. 'Don't rub noses with any grizzlies—shoot 'em, but don't scare 'em to death!'

Jim thumbed his nose as the seaplane speeded up, leaving

a frothy wake. He felt a queer chill as the amphibian took off. For three weeks he would be isolated in this remote valley of the Canadian Rockies. If for any reason the plane failed to return to the icy blue lake, he would surely die. Even with enough food, no man could surmount the frozen peaks and make his way on foot over hundreds of miles of almost virgin wilderness. But of course, Walt Leonard would return on schedule, and it was up to Jim whether or not they lost their stake. If there was any uranium in the valley, he had twenty-one days to find it. To work then, and no gloomy forebodings.

Moving with the unhurried precision of an experienced woodsman, he built a lean-to in the shelter of a rocky overhang. For this three weeks of summer, nothing more permanent was needed. Perspiring in the strong morning sun, he piled his supplies back under the ledge, well covered by a waterproof tarpaulin, and protected from the larger animal prowlers. All but the dynamite: that he cached, also carefully wrapped against moisture, two hundred yards away. Only a fool shares his quarters with a box of high explosives.

The first two weeks went by all too swiftly without any encouraging finds. There was only one good possibility left and just enough time to explore it. So early one morning towards the end of his third week, Jim Irwin prepared for a last-ditch foray into the north-east part of the valley, a region he had not yet visited.

He took the Geiger counter, slipping on the earphones, reversed to keep the normal rattle from dulling his hearing, and reaching for the rifle, set out, telling himself it was now or never so far as this particular expedition was concerned. The bulky .30-06 was a nuisance, and he had no enthusiasm for its weight, but the huge grizzlies of Canada are not intruded upon with impunity, and take a lot of killing. He'd already had to dispose of two, a hateful chore since the big bears were vanishing all too fast. And the rifle had proved a great comfort on several ticklish occasions when actual firing had been avoided. The .22 pistol he left in its sheepskin holster in the lean-to.

He was whistling at the start, for the clear, frosty air, the bright sun on blue-white ice fields, and the heady smell of summer all delighted his heart despite his bad luck as a prospector. He planned to go one day's journey to the new region, spend about thirty-six hours exploring it intensively, and be back in time to meet the plane at noon. Except for his emergency packet, he took no food or water. It would be easy enough to knock over a rabbit, and the streams were alive with firm-fleshed rainbow trout of the kind no longer common in the States.

All morning Jim walked, feeling an occasional surge of hope as the counter chattered. But its clatter always died down. The valley had nothing radioactive of value, only traces. Apparently they'd made a bad choice. His cheerfulness faded. They needed a strike badly, especially Walt. And his own wife, Cele, with a kid on the way. But there was still a chance. These last thirty-six hours he'd snoop at night if necessary—might be the pay-off. He reflected a little bitterly that it would help quite a bit if some of those birds he'd staked would make a strike and return his dough. Right this minute there were close to eight thousand bucks owing to him.

A wry smile touched his lips and he abandoned unprofitable speculations for plans about lunch. The sun, as well as his stomach, said it was time. He had just decided to take out his line and fish a foaming brook, when he rounded a grassy knoll, to come upon a sight that made him stiffen to a halt, his jaw dropping.

It was like some enterprising giant's outdoor butcher shop: a great assortment of animal bodies, neatly lined up in a triple row that extended almost as far as the eye could see. And what animals! To be sure, those nearest him were ordinary deer, bear, cougars and mountain sheep—one of each, apparently—but down the line were strange, uncouth, half-formed hairy beasts; and beyond them a nightmare conglomeration of reptiles. One of the latter, at the extreme end of the remarkable display, he recognized at once. There had been a much larger specimen, fabricated about an incomplete skeleton, of course, in the museum at home.

No doubt about it—it was a small stegosaur, no bigger than a pony!

Fascinated, Jim walked down the line, glancing back over the immense array. Peering more closely at one scaly, dirty-yellow lizard, he saw an eyelid tremble. Then he realized the truth. The animals were not dead but paralysed and miraculously preserved. Perspiration prickled his forehead. How long since stegosaurs had roamed this valley?

All at once he noticed another curious circumstance: the victims were roughly of a size. Nowhere, for example, was there a really large saurian. No tyrannosaurus. For that matter, no mammoth. Each specimen was about the size of a large sheep. He was pondering this odd fact when the underbrush rustled a warning behind him.

Jim Irwin had once worked with mercury, and for a second it seemed to him that a half-filled leather sack of the liquid-metal had rolled into the clearing. For the quasi-spherical object moved with just such a weighty, fluid motion. But it was not leather; and what appeared at first a disgusting wartiness, turned out on closer scrutiny to be more like the functional projections of some outlandish mechanism. Whatever the thing was, he had little time to study it, for after the spheroid had whipped out and retracted a number of metal rods with bulbous, lens-like structures at their tips, it rolled towards him at a speed of about five miles an hour. And from its purposeful advance, the man had no doubt that it meant to add him to the pathetic heap of living-dead specimens.

Uttering an incoherent exclamation, Jim sprang back a number of paces, unslinging his rifle. The ruum that had been left behind was still some thirty yards off, approaching at that moderate but invariable velocity, an advance more terrifying in its regularity than the headlong charge of a mere brute beast.

Jim's hand flew to the bolt, and with practised deftness he slammed a cartridge into the chamber. He snuggled the battered stock against cheek, and using the peep sight, aimed squarely at the leathery bulk—a perfect target in the bright afternoon sun. A grim little smile touched his lips as he squeezed the trigger. He knew what one of those 180-grain, metal-jacketed, boat-tail slugs could do at 2700 feet per second. Probably at this close range it would keyhole and blow the foul thing into a mush, by God!

Wham! The familiar kick against his shoulder. E-e-e-e! The whining screech of a ricochet. He sucked in his breath. There could be no doubt whatever. At a mere twenty yards a bullet from this hard-hitting rifle had glanced from the ruum's surface.

Frantically Jim worked the bolt. He blasted two more rounds, then realized the utter futility of such tactics. When the ruum was six feet away, he saw gleaming fingerhooks flick from warty knobs, and a hollow, sting-like probe dripping greenish liquid, poised snakily between them. The man turned and fled.

Jim Irwin weighed exactly 149 pounds.

It was easy enough to pull ahead. The ruum seemed incapable of increasing its speed. But Jim had no illusions on that score. The steady five-mile-an-hour pace was something no organism on earth could maintain for more than a few hours. Before long, Jim guessed, the hunted animal had either turned on its implacable pursuer, or, in the case of more timid creatures, run itself to exhaustion in a circle out of sheer panic. Only the winged were safe. But for anything on the ground the result was inevitable: another specimen for the awesome array. And for whom the whole collection? Why? Why?

Coolly, as he ran, Jim began to shed all surplus weight. He glanced at the reddening sun, wondering about the coming night. He hesitated over the rifle; it had proved useless against the ruum, but his military training impelled him to keep the weapon to the last. Still, every pound raised the odds against him in the gruelling race he foresaw clearly. Logic told him that military reasoning did not apply to a contest like this; there would be no disgrace in abandoning a worthless rifle. And when weight became really vital, the .30-06 would go. But meanwhile he slung it over one shoulder. The Geiger counter he placed as gently as possible on a flat rock, hardly breaking his stride.

One thing was damned certain. This would be no rabbit run, a blind, panicky flight until exhausted, ending in squealing submission. This would be a fighting retreat, and he'd use every trick of survival he'd learned in his hazard-filled lifetime.

Taking deep measured breaths, he loped along, watching with shrewd eyes for anything that might be used for his advantage in the weird contest. Luckily the valley was sparsely wooded; in brush or forest his straightway speed would be almost useless.

Suddenly he came upon a sight that made him pause. It was a point where a huge boulder overhung the trail, and Jim saw possibilities in the situation. He grinned as he remembered a

Malay mantrap that had once saved his life. Springing to a hillock, he looked back over the grassy plain. The afternoon sun cast long shadows, but it was easy enough to spot the pursuing ruum, still oozing along on Jim's trail. He watched the thing with painful anxiety. Everything hinged upon this brief survey. He was right! Yes, although at most places the man's trail was neither the only route nor the best one, the ruum dogged the footsteps of his prey. The significance of that fact was immense, but Irwin had no more than twelve minutes to implement the knowledge.

Deliberately dragging his feet, Irwin made it a clear trail directly under the boulder. After going past it for about ten yards, he walked backwards in his own prints until just short of the overhang, then jumped up clear of the track to a point behind the balanced rock.

Whipping out his heavy-duty belt knife, he began to dig, scientifically, but with furious haste, about the base of the boulder. Every few moments, sweating with apprehension and effort, he rammed it with one shoulder. At last it teetered a little. He had just jammed the knife back into his sheath and was crouching there, panting, when the ruum rolled into sight over a small ridge on his back trail.

He watched the grey spheroid moving towards him and fought to quiet his sobbing breath. There was no telling what other senses it might bring into play, even though the ruum seemed to prefer just to follow in his prints. But it certainly had a whole battery of instruments at its disposal. He crouched low behind the rock, every nerve a charged wire.

But there was no change of technique by the ruum: seemingly intent on the footprints of its prey, the strange sphere rippled along, passing directly under the great boulder. As it did so Irwin gave a savage yell, and thrusting his whole muscular weight against the balanced mass, toppled it squarely on the ruum. Five tons of stone fell from a height of twelve feet.

Jim scrambled down. He stood there, staring at the huge lump and shaking his head dazedly. 'Fixed that son of a bitch!' he said in a thick voice. He gave the boulder a kick. 'Ha! Walt and I might clear a buck or two yet from your little meat market. Maybe this expedition won't be a total loss. Enjoy yourself in hell where you came from!'

Then he leaped back, his eyes wild. The giant rock was shifting! Slowly its five-ton bulk was sliding off the trail, raising a ridge of soil as it grated along. Even as he stared the boulder tilted, and a grey protuberance appeared under the nearest edge. With a choked cry Jim Irwin broke into a lurching run.

He ran a full mile down the trail. Then finally he stopped and looked back. He could just make out a dark dot moving away from the fallen rock. It progressed as slowly and as regularly and as inexorably as before, and in his direction. Jim sat down heavily, putting his head in his scratched, grimy hands.

But his despairing mood did not last. After all, he had gained a twenty-minute respite. Lying down, trying to relax as much as possible, he took the flat packet of emergency rations from his jacket, and eating quickly but without bolting, disposed of some pemmican, biscuit, and chocolate. A few sips of icy water from a streamlet, and he was almost ready to continue his fantastic struggle. But first he swallowed one of the three benzedrine pills he carried for physical crises. When the ruum was still an estimated ten minutes away, Jim Irwin trotted off, with much of his wiry strength back, and fresh courage to counter bone-deep weariness.

After running for fifteen minutes he came to a sheer face of rock about thirty feet high. The terrain on either side was barely passable, consisting of choked gullies, spiky brush and knife-edged rocks. If Jim could make the top of this little cliff, the ruum surely would have to detour, a circumstance that might put it many minutes behind him.

He looked up at the sun. Huge and crimson, it was almost touching the horizon. He would have to move fast. Irwin was no rock climber but he did know the fundamentals. Using every crevice, roughness, and minute ledge, he fought his way up the cliff. Somehow—unconsciously—he used that flowing climb of a natural mountaineer, which takes each foothold very briefly as an unstressed pivot point in a series of rhythmic advances.

He had just reached the top when the ruum rolled up to the base of the cliff.

Jim knew very well that he ought to leave at once, taking advantage of the few precious remaining moments of daylight. Every second gained was of tremendous value; but curiosity and hope made him wait. He told himself that the instant his pursuer detoured he would get out of there all the faster. Besides, the thing might even give up and he could sleep right here.

Sleep! His body lusted for it.

But the ruum would not detour. It hesitated only a few seconds at the foot of the barrier. Then a number of knobs opened to extrude metallic wands. One of these, topped with lenses, waved in the air. Jim drew back too late—their uncanny gaze had found him as he lay on top of the cliff, peering down. He cursed his idiocy.

Immediately all the wands retracted, and from a different knob a slender rod, blood-red in the setting sun, began to shoot straight up to the man. As he watched, frozen in place, its barbed tip gripped the cliff's edge almost under his nose.

Jim leaped to his feet. Already the rod was shortening as the ruum reabsorbed its shining length. And the leathery sphere was rising off the ground. Swearing loudly, Jim fixed his eyes on the tenacious hook, drawing back one heavy foot.

But experience restrained him. The mighty kick was never launched. He had seen too many rough-and-tumbles lost by an injudicious attempt at the boot. It wouldn't do at all to let any part of his body get within reach of the ruum's superb tools. Instead he seized a length of dry branch, and inserting one end under the metal hook, began to pry.

There was a sputtering flash, white and lacy, and even through the dry wood he felt the potent surge of power that splintered the end. He dropped the smouldering stick with a gasp of pain, and wringing his numb fingers, backed off several steps, full of impotent rage. For a moment he paused, half inclined to run again, but then his upper lip drew back and, snarling, he unslung his rifle. By God! he knew he had been right to lug the damned thing all this way—even if it had beaten a tattoo on his ribs. Now he had the ruum right where he wanted it!

Kneeling to steady his aim in the failing light Jim sighted the hook and fired. There was a soggy thud as the ruum fell. Jim shouted. The heavy slug had done a lot more than he expected. Not only had it blasted the metal claw loose, but it had smashed a big gap in the cliff's edge. It would be pretty damned hard for the ruum to use that part of the rock again!

He looked down. Sure enough, the ruum was back at the

bottom. Jim Irwin grinned. Every time the thing clamped a hook over the bluff, he'd blow that hook loose. There was plenty of ammunition in his pocket and until the moon rose, bringing a good light for shooting with it, he'd stick the gun's muzzle inches away if necessary. Besides, the thing—whatever it might be—was obviously too intelligent to keep up a hopeless struggle. Sooner or later it would accept the detour. And then, maybe the night would help to hide his trail.

Then—he choked, and for a brief moment tears came to his eyes. Down below, in the dimness, the squat, phlegmatic spheroid was extruding three hooked rods simultaneously in a fanlike spread. In a perfectly co-ordinated movement, the rods snagged the cliff's edge at intervals of about four feet.

Jim Irwin whipped the rifle to his shoulder. All right—this was going to be just like the rapid fire for record back at Benning. Only at Benning they didn't expect good shooting in the dark!

But the first shot was a bull's eye, smacking the left-hand hook loose in a puff of rock dust. His second shot did almost as well, knocking the gritty stuff loose so the centre barb slipped off. But even as he whirled to level at number three, Jim saw it was hopeless.

The first hook was back in place. No matter how well he shot, at least one rod would always be in position, pulling the ruum to the top.

Jim hung the useless rifle muzzle down from a stunted tree and ran into the deepening dark. The toughening of his body, a process of years, was paying off now. So what? Where was he going? What could he do now? Was there anything that could stop the damned thing behind him?

Then he remembered the dynamite.

Gradually changing his course, the weary man cut back towards his camp by the lake. Overhead the stars brightened, pointing the way. Jim lost all sense of time. He must have eaten as he wobbled along, for he wasn't hungry. Maybe he could eat at the lean-to . . . no, there wouldn't be time . . . take a benzedrine pill. No, the pills were all gone and the moon was up and he could hear the ruum close behind. Close.

Quite often phosphorescent eyes peered at him from the

underbrush and once, just at dawn, a grizzly whoofed with displeasure at his passage.

Sometimes during the night his wife, Cele, stood before him with outstretched arms. 'Go away!' he rasped. 'Go away! You can make it! It can't chase both of us!' So she turned and ran lightly alongside of him. But when Irwin panted across a tiny glade, Cele faded away into the moonlight and he realized she hadn't been there at all.

Shortly after sunrise Jim Irwin reached the lake. The ruum was close enough for him to hear the dull sounds of its passage. Jim staggered, his eyes closed. He hit himself feebly on the nose, his eyes jerked open, and he saw the explosive. The sight of the greasy sticks of dynamite snapped Irwin wide awake.

He forced himself to calmness and carefully considered what to do. Fuse? No. It would be impossible to leave fused dynamite in the trail and time the detonation with the absolute precision he needed. Sweat poured down his body: his clothes were sodden with it. It was hard to think. The explosion *must* be set off from a distance and at the exact moment the ruum was passing over it. But Irwin dared not use a long fuse. The rate of burning was not constant enough. He couldn't calibrate it perfectly with the ruum's advance. Jim Irwin's body sagged all over, his chin sank toward his heaving chest. He jerked his head up, stepped back—and saw the .22 pistol where he had left it in the lean-to.

His sunken eyes flashed.

Moving with frenetic haste, he took the half-filled case, piled all the remaining percussion caps among the loose sticks in a devil's mixture. Weaving out to the trail, he carefully placed box and contents directly on his earlier tracks some twenty yards from a rocky ledge. It was a risk—the stuff might go any time—but that didn't matter. He would far rather be blown to rags than end up living but paralysed in the ruum's outdoor butcher's stall.

The exhausted Irwin had barely hunched down behind the thin ledge of rock before his inexorable pursuer appeared over a slight rise five hundred yards away. Jim scrunched deeper into the hollow, then saw a vertical gap, a narrow crack between rocks. That was it, he thought vaguely. He could sight through the gap at the dynamite and still be shielded from the blast. If it was a shield . . . when that half-case blew only twenty yards away . . .

He stretched out on his belly, watching the ruum roll forward. A hammer of exhaustion pounded his ballooning skull. When had he slept last? This was the first time he had lain down in hours. Hours? Ha! It was days. His muscles stiffened, locked into throbbing, burning knots. Then he felt the morning sun on his back, soothing, warming, easing . . . No! If he let go, if he slept now, it was the ruum's macabre collection for Jim Irwin! Stiff fingers tightened around the pistol. He'd stay awake! If he lost—if the ruum survived the blast—there'd still be time to put a bullet through his brain.

He looked down at the sleek pistol, then out at the innocent-seeming booby trap. If he timed this right—and he would—the ruum wouldn't survive. No. He relaxed a little, yielding just a bit to the gently insistent sun. A bird whistled softly somewhere above him and a fish splashed in the lake.

Suddenly he was wrenched to full awareness. Damn! Of all times for a grizzly to come snooping about! With the whole of Irwin's camp ready for greedy looting, a fool bear had to come sniffing around the dynamite! The furred monster smelled carefully at the box, nosed around, rumbled deep displeasure at the alien scent of man. Irwin held his breath. Just a touch would blow a cap. A single cap meant . . .

The grizzly lifted his head from the box and growled hoarsely. The box was ignored, the offensive odour of man was forgotten. Its feral little eyes focused on a plodding spheroid that was now only forty yards away. Jim Irwin snickered. Until he had met the ruum the grizzly bear of the North American continent was the only thing in the world he had ever feared. And now—why the hell was he so calm about it?—the two terrors of his existence were meeting head on and he was laughing. He shook his head and the great side muscles in his neck hurt abominably. He looked down at his pistol, then out at the dynamite. *These* were the only real things in his world.

About six feet from the bear, the ruum paused. Still in the grip of that almost idiotic detachment, Jim Irwin found himself wondering again what it was, where it had come from. The grizzly arose on its haunches, the embodiment of utter ferocity. Terrible teeth flashed white against red lips. The business-like ruum started to roll past. The bear closed in, roaring. It cuffed at the ruum. A mighty paw, armed with black claws sharper and stronger than scythes, made that cuff. It would have disembowelled a rhinoceros. Irwin cringed as that side-swipe knocked dust from the leathery sphere. The ruum was hurled back several inches. It paused, recovered, and with the same dreadful casualness it rippled on, making a wider circle, ignoring the bear.

But the lord of the woods wasn't settling for any draw. Moving with that incredible agility which has terrified Indians, Spanish, French and Anglo-Americans since the first encounter of any of them with his species, the grizzly whirled, sidestepped beautifully, and hugged the ruum. The terrible, shaggy forearms tightened, the slavering jaws champed at the grey surface. Irwin half rose. 'Go it!' he croaked. Even as he cheered the clumsy emperor of the wild, Jim thought it was an insane tableau: the village idiot wrestling with a beach ball.

Then silver metal gleamed brightly against grey. There was a flash, swift and deadly. The roar of the king abruptly became a whimper, a gurgle, and then there was nearly a ton of terror wallowing in death—its throat slashed open. Jim Irwin saw the bloody blade retract into the grey spheroid, leaving a bright-red smear on the thing's dusty hide.

And the ruum rolled forward past the giant corpse, implacable, still intent on the man's spoor, his footprints, his pathway. Okay, baby, Jim giggled at the dead grizzly, this is for you, for Cele, for lots of poor dumb animals like us—come to, you damned fool, he cursed at himself. And aimed at the dynamite. And very calmly, very carefully, Jim Irwin squeezed the trigger of his pistol.

Briefly, sound first. Then giant hands lifted his body from where he lay, then let go. He came down hard, face in a patch of nettles, but he was sick, he didn't care. He remembered that the birds were quiet. Then there was a fluid thump as something massive struck the grass a few yards away. Then there was quiet.

Irwin lifted his head . . . all men do in such a case. His body still ached. He lifted sore shoulders and saw . . . an enormous, smoking crater in the earth. He also saw, a dozen paces away, grey-white because it was covered now with powdered rock, the ruum.

It was under a tall, handsome pine tree. Even as Jim watched, wondering if the ringing in his ears would ever stop, the ruum rolled towards him.

Irwin fumbled for his pistol. It was gone. It had dropped somewhere out of reach. He wanted to pray then, but couldn't get properly started. Instead, he kept thinking idiotically, 'My sister Ethel can't spell Nebuchadnezzar and never could. My sister Ethel—'

The ruum was a foot away now, and Jim closed his eyes. He felt cool, metallic fingers touch, grip, lift. His unresisting body was raised several inches and juggled oddly. Shuddering, he waited for the terrible syringe with its green liquid, seeing the yellow, shrunken face of a lizard with one eyelid a-tremble.

Then, dispassionately, without either roughness or solicitude, the ruum put him back on the ground. When he opened his eyes, some seconds later, the sphere was rolling away. Watching it go, he sobbed dryly.

It seemed a matter of moments only before he heard the seaplane's engine, and opened his eyes to see Walt Leonard bending over him.

Later, in the plane, five thousand feet above the valley, Walt grinned suddenly, slapped him on the back, and cried: 'Jim, I can get a whirlybird, a four-place job! Why, if we can snatch up just a few of those prehistoric lizards and things while the museum keeper's away, it's like you said—the scientists will pay us plenty.'

Jim's hollow eyes lit up. 'That's the idea,' he agreed.

Then bitterly: 'I might just as well have stayed in bed. Evidently the damned thing didn't want me at all. Maybe it wanted to know what I paid for these pants! Barely touched me, then let go. And how I ran!'

'Yeah,' Walt said. 'That was damned queer. And after that marathon. I admire your guts, boy.' He glanced sideways at Jim Irwin's haggard face. 'That night's run cost you plenty. I figure you lost over ten pounds.'

Through the Tunnel *by Doris Lessing*

Going to the shore on the first morning of the holiday, the young English boy stopped at a turning of the path and looked down at a wild and rocky bay, and then over to the crowded beach he knew so well from other years. His mother walked on in front of him, carrying a bright-striped bag in one hand. Her other arm, swinging loose, was very white in the sun. The boy watched that white, naked arm, and turned his eyes, which had a frown behind them, toward the bay and back again to his mother. When she felt he was not with her, she swung around. 'Oh, there you are Jerry!' she said. She looked impatient, then smiled. 'Why, darling, would you rather not come with me? Would you rath—' She frowned, conscientiously worrying over what amusements he might secretly be longing for which she had been too busy or too careless to imagine. He was very familiar with that anxious, apologetic smile. Contrition sent him running after her. And yet, as he ran, he looked back over his shoulder at the wild bay; and all morning, as he played on the safe beach, he was thinking of it.

Next morning, when it was time for the routine of swimming and sunbathing, his mother said, 'Are you tired of the usual beach, Jerry? Would you like to go somewhere else?'

'Oh, no!' he said quickly, smiling at her out of that unfailing impulse of contrition—a sort of chivalry. Yet, walking down the path with her, he blurted out, 'I'd like to go and have a look at those rocks down there.'

She gave the idea her attention. It was a wild-looking place, and there was no-one there, but she said, 'Of course, Jerry. When you've had enough, come to the big beach. Or just go straight back to the villa, if you like.' She walked away, that bare arm, now slightly reddened from yesterday's sun, swinging. And he almost ran after her again, feeling it unbearable that she should go by herself, but he did not.

She was thinking, of course he's old enough to be safe without me. Have I been keeping him too close? He mustn't feel he ought to be with me. I must be careful.

Through the Tunnel

He was an only child, eleven years old. She was a widow. She was determined to be neither possessive nor lacking in devotion. She went worrying off to her beach.

As for Jerry, once he saw that his mother had gained her beach, he began the steep descent to the bay. From where he was, high up among red-brown rocks, it was a scoop of moving bluish-green fringed with white. As he went lower, he saw that it spread among small promontories and inlets of rough, sharp rock, and the crisping, lapping surface showed stains of purple and darker blue. Finally, as he ran sliding and scraping down the last few yards, he saw an edge of white surf, and the shallow, luminous movement of water over white sand, and beyond that, a solid, heavy blue.

He ran straight into the water and began swimming. He was a good swimmer. He went out fast over the gleaming sand, over a middle region where rocks lay like discoloured monsters under the surface, and then he was in the real sea—a warm sea where irregular cold currents from the deep water shocked his limbs.

When he was so far out that he could look back not only on the little bay but past the promontory that was between it and the big beach, he floated on the buoyant surface and looked for his mother. There she was, a speck of yellow under an umbrella that looked like a slice of orange peel. He swam back to shore, relieved at being sure she was there, but all at once very lonely.

On the edge of a small cape that marked the side of the bay away from the promontory was a loose scatter of rocks. Above them, some boys were stripping off their clothes. They came running, naked, down to the rocks. The English boy swam towards them and kept his distance at a stone's throw. They were of that coast, all of them burned smooth dark brown, and speaking a language he did not understand. To be with them, of them, was a craving that filled his whole body. He swam a little closer; they turned and watched him with narrowed alert dark eyes. Then one smiled and waved. It was enough. In a minute he had swum in and was on the rocks beside them, smiling with a desperate, nervous supplication. They shouted cheerful greetings at him, and then, as he preserved his nervous, uncomprehending smile, they understood that he was a foreigner strayed from his own beach, and they proceeded to forget him. But he was happy. He was with them.

They began diving again and again from a high point into a well of blue sea between rough, pointed rocks. After they had dived and come up, they swam around, hauled themselves up, and waited their turn to dive again. They were big boys—men to Jerry. He dived, and they watched him, and when he swam around to take his place, they made way for him. He felt he was accepted, and he dived again, carefully proud of himself.

Soon the biggest of the boys poised himself, shot down into the water, and did not come up. The others stood about, watching. Jerry, after waiting for the sleek brown head to appear, let out a yell of warning; they looked at him idly and turned their eyes back towards the water. After a long time, the boy came up on the other side of a big dark rock, letting the air out of his lungs in a sputtering gasp and a shout of triumph. Immediately, the rest of them dived in. One moment, the morning seemed full of chattering boys; the next, the air and the surface of the water were empty. But through the heavy blue, dark shapes could be seen moving and groping.

Jerry dived, shot past the school of underwater swimmers, saw a black wall of rock looming at him, touched it, and bobbed up at once to the surface, where the wall was a low barrier he could see across. There was no-one visible; under him, in the water, the dim shapes of the swimmers had disappeared. Then one, and then another of the boys came up on the far side of the barrier of rock, and he understood that they had swum through some gap or hole in it. He plunged down again. He could see nothing through the stinging salt water but the blank rock. When he came up the boys were all on the diving rock preparing to attempt the feat again. And now, in a panic of failure, he yelled up, in English, 'Look at me! Look!' and he began splashing and kicking in the water like a foolish dog.

They looked down gravely, frowning. He knew the frown. At moments of failure, when he clowned to claim his mother's attention, it was with just this grave, embarrassed inspection that she rewarded him. Through his hot shame, feeling the pleading grin on his face like a scar that he could never remove, he looked up at the group of big brown boys on the rock and shouted, '*Bonjour! Merci! Au revoir! Monsieur, monsieur!*' while he hooked his fingers round his ears and waggled them.

Water surged into his mouth; he choked, sank, came up. The rock, lately weighted with boys, seemed to rear up out of the water as their weight was removed. They were flying down past him now, into the water: the air was full of falling bodies. Then the rock was empty in the hot sunlight. He counted one, two, three . . .

At fifty, he was terrified. They must all be drowning beneath him, in the watery caves of the rock! At a hundred, he stared around him at the empty hillside, wondering if he should yell for help. He counted faster, faster, to hurry them up, to bring them to the surface quickly, to drown them quickly—anything rather than the terror of counting on and on into the blue emptiness of the morning. And then, at a hundred and sixty, the water beyond the rock was full of boys blowing like brown whales. They swam back to the shore without a look at him.

He climbed back to the diving rock and sat down, feeling the hot roughness of it under his thighs. The boys were gathering up their bits of clothing and running off along the shore to another promontory. They were leaving to get away from him. He cried openly, fists in his eyes. There was no-one to see him, and he cried himself out.

It seemed to him that a long time had passed, and he swam out to where he could see his mother. Yes, she was still there, a yellow spot under an orange umbrella. He swam back to the big rock, climbed up, and dived into the blue pool among the fanged and angry boulders. Down he went, until he touched the wall of rock again. But the salt was so painful in his eyes that he could not see.

He came to the surface, swam to shore and went back to the villa to wait for his mother. Soon she walked slowly up the path, swinging her striped bag, the flushed naked arm dangling beside her. 'I want some swimming goggles,' he panted, defiant and beseeching.

She gave him a patient, inquisitive look as she said casually, 'Well, of course, darling.'

But now, now, now! He must have them this minute and no other time. He nagged and pestered until she went with him to a shop. As soon as she had bought the goggles, he grabbed them from her hand as if she were going to claim them for herself, and was off, running down the steep path to the bay.

Jerry swam out to the big barrier rock, adjusted the goggles, and dived. The impact of the water broke the rubber-enclosed vacuum, and the goggles came loose. He understood that he must swim down to the base of the rock from the surface of the water. He fixed the goggles tight and firm, filled his lungs, and floated face down on the water. Now he could see. It was as if he had eyes of a different kind—fish-eyes that showed everything clear and delicate and wavering in the bright water.

Under him, six or seven feet down, was a floor of perfectly clean, shining white sand, rippled firm and hard by the tides. Two greyish shapes steered there, like long, rounded pieces of wood or slate. They were fish. He saw them nose towards each other, poise motionless, make a dart forward, swerve off and come around again. It was like a water dance. A few inches above them, the water sparkled as if sequins were dropping through it. Fish again—myriads of minute fish, the length of his fingernail, were drifting through the water, and in a moment he could feel the innumerable tiny touches of them against his limbs. It was like swimming in flaked silver. The great rock the big boys had swum through rose sheer out of the white sand, black, tufted lightly with greenish weed. He could see no gap in it. He swam down to its base.

Again and again he rose, took a big chestful of air, and went down. Again and again he groped over the surface of the rock, feeling it, almost hugging it in the desperate need to find the entrance. And then once, while he was clinging to the black wall, his knees came up and he shot his feet out forward and they met no obstacle. He had found the hole.

He gained the surface, clambered about the stones that littered the barrier rock until he found a big one, and with this in his arms let himself down over the side of the rock. He dropped with the weight straight to the sandy floor. Clinging tight to the anchor of stone, he lay on his side and looked in under the dark shelf at the place where his feet had gone. He could see the hole. It was an irregular, dark gap, but he could not see deep into it. He let go of his anchor, clung with his hands to the edges of the hole, and tried to push himself in.

He got his head in, found his shoulders jammed, moved them in sidewise, and was inside as far as his waist. He could see nothing ahead. Something soft and clammy touched his mouth, he saw a dark frond moving against the greyish rock, and panic filled him. He thought of octopuses, of clinging weed. He pushed himself out backwards and caught a glimpse, as he retreated, of a harmless tentacle of seaweed drifting in the mouth of the tunnel. But it was enough. He reached the sunlight, swam to shore, and lay on the diving rock. He looked down into the blue well of water. He knew he must find his way through the cave, or hole, or tunnel, and out the other side.

First, he thought, he must learn to control his breathing. He let himself down into the water with another big stone in his arms, so that he could lie effortlessly on the bottom of the sea. He counted. One, two, three. He counted steadily. He could hear the movement of blood in his chest. Fifty-one, fifty-two . . . His chest was hurting. He let go of the rock and went up into the air. He saw that the sun was low. He rushed to the villa and found his mother at her supper. She said only, 'Did you enjoy yourself?' and he said, 'Yes.'

All night the boy dreamed of the water-filled cave in the rock, and as soon as breakfast was over he went to the bay.

That night his nose bled badly. For hours he had been underwater, learning to hold his breath, and now he felt weak and dizzy. His mother said, 'I shouldn't overdo things, darling, if I were you.'

That day and the next Jerry exercised his lungs as if everything, the whole of his life, all that he would become, depended upon it. And again his nose bled at night, and his mother insisted on his coming with her the next day. It was a torment to him to waste a day of his careful self-training, but he stayed with her on that other beach, which now seemed a place for small children, a place where his mother might lie safe in the sun. It was not his beach.

He did not ask for permission on the following day to go to his beach. He went before his mother could consider the complicated rights and wrongs of the matter. A day's rest, he discovered, had improved his count by ten. The big boys had made the passage while he counted a hundred and sixty. He had been counting fast in his fright. Probably now, if he tried, he could get through that long tunnel, but he was not going to try yet. A curious, most unchildlike persistence, a controlled impatience, made him wait. In the meantime he lay underwater on the white sand, littered now by stones he had brought down from the upper air, and studied the entrance to the tunnel. He knew every jut and corner of it, as far as it was possible to see. It was as if he already felt its sharpness about his shoulders.

He sat by the clock in the villa when his mother was not near, and checked his time. He was incredulous and then proud to find that he could hold his breath without strain for two minutes. The words 'two minutes', authorized by the clock, brought the adventure that was so necessary to him close.

In another four days, his mother said casually one morning, they must go home. On the day before they left, he would do it. He would do it if it killed him, he said defiantly to himself. But two days before they were to leave—a day of triumph when he increased his count by fifteen—his nose bled so badly that he turned dizzy and had to lie limply over the big rock like a bit of seaweed, watching the thick red blood flow on to the rock and trickle slowly down to the sea. He was frightened. Supposing he turned dizzy in the tunnel? Supposing he died there, trapped? Supposing—his head went around in the hot sun, and he almost gave up. He thought he would return to the house and lie down, and next summer, perhaps, when he had another year's growth in him—then he would go through the hole.

But even after he had made the decision, or thought he had, he found himself sitting up on the rock and looking down into the water, and he knew that now, this moment, when his nose had only just stopped bleeding, when his head was still sore and throbbing—this was the moment when he would try. If he did not do it now, he never would. He was trembling with fear that he would not go, and he was trembling with horror at that long, long tunnel under the rock, under the sea. Even in the open sunlight the barrier rock seemed very wide and very heavy; tons of rock pressed down on where he would go. If he died there, he would lie until one day—perhaps not before next year—those big boys would swim into it and find it blocked.

He put on his goggles, fitted them tight, tested the vacuum. His hands were shaking. Then he chose the biggest stone he could carry and slipped over the edge of the rock until half of him was in the cool, enclosing water and half in the hot sun. He looked up once at the empty sky, filled his lungs once, twice, and then sank fast to the bottom with the stone. He let it go and began to count. He took the edges of the hole in his hands and drew himself into it, wriggling his shoulders in sidewise as he remembered he must, kicking himself along with his feet.

Soon he was clear inside. He was in a small rock-bound hole filled with yellowish-grey water. The water was pushing him up against the roof. The roof was sharp and pained his back. He pulled himself along with his hands—fast, fast—and used his legs as levers. His head knocked against something; a sharp pain dizzied him. Fifty, fifty-one, fifty-two . . . He was without light, and the water seemed to press upon him with the weight of the rock. Seventy-one, seventy-two . . . There was no strain on his lungs. He felt like an inflated balloon, his lungs were so light and easy, but his head was pulsing.

He was being continually pressed against the sharp roof, which felt slimy as well as sharp. Again he thought of octopuses, and wondered if the tunnel might be filled with weed that could tangle him. He gave himself a panicky convulsive kick forward, ducked his head, and swam. His feet and hands moved freely, as if in open water. The hole must have widened out. He thought he must be swimming fast, and he was frightened of banging his head if the tunnel narrowed.

A hundred, a hundred and one . . . The water paled. Victory filled him. His lungs were beginning to hurt. A few more strokes and he would be out. He was counting wildly; he said a hundred and fifteen, and then a long time later, a hundred and fifteen again. The water was a clear jewel-green all around him. Then he saw, above his head, a crack running up through the rock. Sunlight was falling through it, showing the clean dark rock of the tunnel, a single mussel shell, and darkness ahead.

He was at the end of what he could do. He looked up at the

crack as if it were filled with air and not water, as if he could put his mouth to it to draw in air. A hundred and fifteen, he heard himself say inside his head—but he had said that long ago. He must go on into the blackness ahead or he would drown. His head was swelling, his lungs cracking. A hundred and fifteen, a hundred and fifteen pounded through his head, and he feebly clutched at rocks in the dark, pulling himself forward, leaving the brief space of sunlit water behind. He felt he was dying. He was no longer quite conscious. He struggled on in the darkness between lapses into unconsciousness. An immense, swelling pain filled his head, and then the darkness cracked with an explosion of green light. His hands groping forward, met nothing, and his feet, kicking back, propelled him out into the open sea.

He drifted to the surface, his face turned up to the air. He was gasping like a fish. He felt he would sink now and drown; he could not swim the few feet back to the rock. Then he was clutching it and pulling himself up onto it. He lay face down, gasping. He could see nothing but a red-veined, clotted dark. His eyes must have burst he thought: they were full of blood. He tore off his goggles and a gout of blood went into the sea. His nose was bleeding, and the blood had filled the goggles.

He scooped up handfuls of water from the cool, salty sea to splash on his face, and did not know whether it was blood or salt water he tasted. After a time his heart quieted, his eyes cleared, and he sat up. He could see the local boys diving and playing half a mile away. He did not want them. He wanted nothing but to get back home and lie down.

In a short while Jerry swam to shore and climbed slowly up the path to the villa. He flung himself on his bed and slept, waking at the sound of feet on the path outside. His mother was coming back. He rushed to the bathroom, thinking she must not see his face with blood or tearstains on it. He came out of the bathroom and met her as she walked into the villa, smiling, her eyes lighting up.

'Have a nice morning?' she asked, laying her hand on his warm brown shoulder a moment.

'Oh yes, thank you,' he said.

'You look a bit pale.' And then, sharp and anxious, 'How did you bang your head?'

'Oh, just banged it,' he told her.

She looked at him closely. He was strained. His eyes were glazed-looking. She was worried. And then she said to herself, 'Oh, don't fuss! Nothing can happen. He can swim like a fish.'

They sat down to lunch together.

'Mummy,' he said, 'I can stay underwater for two minutes—three minutes, at least.' It came bursting out of him.

'Can you, darling?' she said. 'Well, I shouldn't overdo it. I don't think you ought to swim any more today.'

She was ready for a battle of wills, but he gave in at once. It was no longer of the least importance to go to the bay.

A Man Called Horse

by Dorothy M Johnson

He was a young man of good family, as the phrase went in the New England of a hundred-odd years ago, and the reasons for his bitter discontent were unclear, even to himself. He grew up in the gracious old Boston home under his grandmother's care, for his mother had died in giving him birth; and all his life he had known every comfort and privilege his father's wealth could provide.

But still there was the discontent, which puzzled him because he could not even define it. He wanted to live among his equals—people who were no better than he and no worse either. That was as close as he could come to describing the source of his unhappiness in Boston and his restless desire to go somewhere else.

In the year 1845 he left home and went out West, far beyond the country's creeping frontier, where he hoped to find his equals. He had the idea that in Indian country, where there was danger, all white men were kings, and he wanted to be one of them. But he found, in the West as in Boston, that the men he respected were still his superiors, even if they could not read, and those he did not respect weren't worth talking to.

He did have money, however, and he could hire the men he respected. He hired four of them, to cook and hunt and guide and be his companions, but he found them not friendly.

They were apart from him and he was still alone. He still brooded about his status in the world, longing for his equals.

On a day in June he learned what it was to have no status at all. He became a captive of a small raiding party of Crow Indians.

He heard gunfire and the brief shouts of his companions around the bend of the creek just before they died, but he never saw their bodies. He had no chance to fight because he was naked and unarmed, bathing in the creek, when a Crow warrior seized and held him.

His captor let him go at last, let him run. Then the lot of them rode him down for sport, striking him with their coup sticks. They carried the dripping scalps of his companions, and one had skinned off Baptiste's black beard as well, for a trophy.

They took him along in a matter-of-fact way, as they took the captured horses. He was unshod and naked as the horses were, and like them he had a rawhide thong around his neck. So long as he didn't fall down, the Crows ignored him.

On the second day they gave him his breeches. His feet were too swollen for his boots, but one of the Indians threw him a pair of moccasins that had belonged to the halfbreed, Henri, who was dead back at the creek. The captive wore the moccasins gratefully. The third day they let him ride one of the spare horses so the party could move faster, and on that day they came in sight of their camp.

He thought of trying to escape, hoping he might be killed in flight rather than by slow torture in the camp, but he never had a chance to try. They were more familiar with escape than he was and, knowing what to expect, they forestalled it. The only other time he had tried to escape from anyone, he had succeeded. When he had left his home in Boston, his father had raged and his grandmother had cried, but they could not talk him out of his intention.

The men of the Crow raiding party didn't bother with talk.

Before riding into camp they stopped and dressed in their regalia, and in parts of their victims' clothing; they painted their faces black. Then, leading the white man by the rawhide around his neck as though he were a horse, they rode down towards the tepee circle, shouting and singing, brandishing their weapons. He was unconscious when they got there; he fell and was dragged.

He lay dazed and battered near a tepee while the noisy, busy life of the camp swarmed around him and Indians came to stare. Thirst consumed him, and when it rained he lapped rainwater from the ground like a dog. A scrawny, shrieking, eternally busy old woman with ragged greying hair threw a chunk of meat on the grass, and he fought the dogs for it.

When his head cleared, he was angry, although anger was an emotion he knew he could not afford.

It was better when I was a horse, he thought—when they

led me by the rawhide around my neck. I won't be a dog, no matter what.

The hag gave him stinking, rancid grease and let him figure out what it was for. He applied it gingerly to his bruised and sun-seared body.

Now, he thought, I smell like the rest of them.

While he was healing, he considered coldly the advantages of being a horse. A man would be humiliated, and sooner or later he would strike back and that would be the end of him. But a horse had only to be docile. Very well, he would learn to do without pride.

He understood that he was the property of the screaming old woman, a fine gift from her son, one that she liked to show off. She did more yelling at him than at anyone else, probably to impress the neighbours so they would not forget what a great and generous man her son was. She was bossy and proud, a dreadful sag of skin and bones, and she was a devilish hard worker.

The white man, who now thought of himself as a horse, forgot sometimes to worry about his danger. He kept making mental notes of things to tell his own people in Boston about this hideous adventure. He would go back a hero, and he would say, 'Grandmother, let me fetch your shawl. I've been accustomed to doing little errands for another lady about your age.'

Two girls lived in the tepee with the old hag and her warrior son. One of them, the white man concluded, was his captor's wife and the other was his little sister. The daughter-in-law was smug and spoiled. Being beloved, she did not have to be useful. The younger girl had bright, wandering eyes. Often enough they wandered to the white man who was pretending to be a horse.

The two girls worked when the old woman put them at it, but they were always running off to do something they enjoyed more. There were games and noisy contests, and there was much laughter. But not for the white man. He was finding out what loneliness could be.

That was a rich summer on the plains, with plenty of buffalo for meat and clothing and the making of tepees. The Crows were wealthy in horses, prosperous and contented. If their men had not been so avid for glory, the white man thought, there would have been a lot more of them. But they went out of their way to court death, and when one of them met it, the whole camp mourned extravagantly and cried to their God for vengeance.

The captive was a horse all summer, a docile bearer of burdens, careful and patient. He kept reminding himself that he had to be better-natured than other horses, because he could not lash out with hoofs or teeth. Helping the old woman load up the horses for travel, he yanked at a pack and said, 'Whoa, brother. It goes easier when you don't fight.'

The horse gave him a big-eyed stare as if it understood his language—a comforting thought, because nobody else did. But even among the horses he felt unequal. They were able to look out for themselves if they escaped. He would simply starve. He was envious still, even among the horses.

Humbly he fetched and carried. Sometimes he even offered to help, but he had not the skill for the endless work of the women, and he was not trusted to hunt with the men, the providers.

When the camp moved he carried a pack, trudging with the women. Even the dogs worked then, pulling small burdens on travois of sticks.

The Indian who had captured him lived like a lord, as he had a right to do. He hunted with his peers, attended long ceremonial meetings with much chanting and dancing, and lounged in the shade with his smug bride. He had only two responsibilities: to kill buffalo and to gain glory. The white man was so far beneath him in status that the Indian did not even think of envy.

One day several things happened that made the captive think he might sometime become a man again. That was the day when he began to understand their language. For four months he had heard it, day and night, the joy and the mourning, the ritual chanting and sung prayers, the squabbles and the deliberations. None of it meant anything to him at all.

But on that important day in early fall the two young women set out for the river, and one of them called over her shoulder to the old woman. The white man was startled. She had said she was going to bathe. His understanding was so sudden that he felt as if his ears had come unstopped. Listening to the racket of the camp, he heard fragments of meaning instead of gabble.

On that same important day the old woman brought a pair of new moccasins out of the tepee and tossed them on the ground before him. He could not believe she would do anything for him because of kindness, but giving him moccasins was one way of looking after her property.

In thanking her, he dared greatly. He picked a little handful of fading fall flowers and took them to her as she squatted in front of her tepee, scraping a buffalo hide with a tool made from a piece of iron tied to a bone. Her hands were hideous—most of the fingers had the first joint missing. He bowed solemnly and offered the flowers.

She glared at him from beneath the short, ragged tangle of her hair. She stared at the flowers, knocked them out of his hand and went running to the next tepee, squalling the story. He heard her and the other women screaming with laughter.

The white man squared his shoulders and walked boldly over to watch three small boys shooting arrows at a target. He said in English, 'Show me how to do that, will you?'

They frowned, but he held out his hand as if there could be no doubt. One of them gave him a bow and one arrow, and they snickered when he missed.

The people were easily amused, except when they were angry. They were amused at him, playing with the little boys. A few days later he asked the hag, with gestures, for a bow that her son had just discarded, a man-sized bow of horn. He scavenged for old arrows. The old woman cackled at his marksmanship and called her neighbours to enjoy the fun.

When he could understand words, he could identify his people by their names. The old woman was Greasy Hand, and her daughter was Pretty Calf. The other young woman's name was not clear to him, for the words were not in his vocabulary. The man who had captured him was Yellow Robe.

Once he could understand, he could begin to talk a little, and then he was less lonely. Nobody had been able to see any reason for talking to him, since he would not understand anyway. He asked the old woman, 'What is my name?' Until he knew it, he was incomplete. She shrugged to let him know he had none.

He told her in the Crow language, 'My name is Horse.' He repeated it, and she nodded. After that they called him Horse when they called him anything. Nobody cared except the white man himself.

They trusted him enough to let him stray out of camp, so that he might have got away and, by unimaginable good luck, reached a trading post or a fort, but winter was too close. He did not dare leave without a horse; he needed clothing and a better hunting weapon than he had, and more certain skill in using it. He did not dare steal, for then they would surely have pursued him, and just as certainly they would have caught him. Remembering the warmth of the home that was waiting in Boston, he settled down for the winter.

On a cold night he crept into the tepee after the others had gone to bed. Even a horse might try to find shelter from the wind. The old woman grumbled, but without conviction. She did not put him out.

They tolerated him, back in the shadows, so long as he did not get in the way.

He began to understand how the family that owned him differed from the others. Fate had been cruel to them. In a short, sharp argument among the old women, one of them derided Greasy Hand by sneering, 'You have no relatives!' and Greasy Hand raved for minutes of the deeds of her father and uncles and brothers. And she had had four sons, she reminded her detractor—who answered with scorn, 'Where are they?'

Later the white man found her moaning and whimpering to herself, rocking back and forth on her haunches, staring at her mutilated hands. By that time he understood. A mourner often chopped off a finger joint. Old Greasy Hand had mourned often. For the first time he felt a twinge of pity, but he put it aside as another emotion, like anger, that he could not afford. He thought: what tales I will tell when I get home.

He wrinkled his nose in disdain. The camp stank of animals and meat and rancid grease. He looked down at his naked, shivering legs and was startled, remembering that he was still only a horse.

He could not trust the old woman. She fed him only because a starved slave would die and not be worth boasting about. Just how fitful her temper was he saw on the day when she got tired of stumbling over one of the hundred dogs that infested the camp. This was one of her own dogs, a large, strong one that pulled a baggage travois when the tribe moved camp.

Countless times he had seen her kick at the beast as it lay sleeping in front of the tepee, in her way. The dog always moved, with a yelp, but it always got in the way again. One day she gave the dog its usual kick and then stood scolding at it while the animal rolled its eyes sleepily. The old woman suddenly picked up her axe and cut the dog's head off with one blow. Looking well satisfied with herself, she beckoned her slave to remove the body.

It could have been me, he thought, if I were a dog. But I'm a horse.

His hope of life lay with the girl, Pretty Calf. He set about courting her, realizing how desperately poor he was both in property and honour. He owned no horse, no weapon but the old bow and the battered arrows. He had nothing to give away, and he needed gifts, because he did not dare seduce the girl.

One of the customs of courtship involved sending a gift of horses to a girl's older brother and bestowing much buffalo meat upon her mother. The white man could not wait for some far-off time when he might have either horses or meat to give away. And his courtship had to be secret. It was not for him to stroll past the groups of watchful girls, blowing a flute made of an eagle's wing bone, as the flirtatious young bucks did.

He could not ride past Pretty Calf's tepee, painted and bedizened: he had no horse, no finery.

Back home, he remembered, I could marry just about any girl I'd wanted to. But he wasted little time thinking about that. A future was something to be earned.

The most he dared do was wink at Pretty Calf now and then, or state his admiration while she giggled and hid her face. The least he dared do to win his bride was to elope with her, but he had to give her a horse to put the seal of tribal approval on that. And he had no horse until he killed a man to get one . . .

His opportunity came in early spring. He was casually accepted by that time. He did not belong, but he was amusing to the Crows, like a strange pet, or they would not have fed him through the winter.

His chance came when he was hunting small game with three young boys who were his guards as well as his scornful companions. Rabbits and birds were of no account in a camp well fed on buffalo meat, but they made good targets.

His party walked far that day. All of them at once saw the two horses in a sheltered coulee. The boys and the man crawled forward on their bellies, and then they saw an Indian who lay on the ground, moaning, a lone traveller. From the way the boys inched eagerly forward, Horse knew the man was fair prey—a member of some enemy tribe.

This is the way the captive white man acquired wealth and honour to win a bride and save his life: he shot an arrow into the sick man, a split second ahead of one of his small companions, and dashed forward to strike the still-groaning man with his bow, to count first coup. Then he seized the hobbled horses.

By the time he had the horses secure and with them his hope for freedom, the boys had followed, counting coup with gestures and shrieks they had practised since boyhood, and one of them had the scalp. The white man was grimly amused to see the boy double up with sudden nausea when he had the thing in his hand . . .

There was a hubbub in the camp when they rode in that evening, two of them on each horse. The captive was noticed. Indians who had ignored him as a slave stared at the brave man who had struck first coup and had stolen horses.

The hubbub lasted all night, as fathers boasted loudly of their young sons' exploits. The white man was called upon to settle an argument between two fierce boys as to which of them had struck second coup and which must be satisfied with third. After much talk that went over his head, he solemnly pointed at the nearest boy. He didn't know which boy it was and didn't care, but the boy did.

The white man had watched warriors in their triumph. He knew what to do. Modesty about achievements had no place among the Crow people. When a man did something big, he told about it.

The white man smeared his face with grease and charcoal. He walked inside the tepee circle, chanting and singing. He used his own language.

'You heathens, you savages,' he shouted. 'I'm going to get out of here someday! I am going to get away!' The Crow people listened respectfully. In the Crow tongue he shouted, 'Horse! I am Horse!' and they nodded.

He had a right to boast and he had two horses. Before dawn the white man and his bride were sheltered beyond a far hill, and he was telling her, 'I love you, little lady. I love you.'

She looked at him with her great dark eyes, and he thought she understood his English words—or as much as she needed to understand.

'You are my treasure,' he said, 'more precious than jewels, better than fine gold. I am going to call you Freedom.'

When they returned to camp two days later, he was bold but worried. His ace, he suspected, might not be high enough in the game he was playing without being sure of the rules. But it served.

Old Greasy Hand raged—but not at him. She complained loudly that her daughter had let herself go too cheap. But the marriage was as good as any Crow marriage. He had paid a horse.

He learned the language faster after that, from Pretty Calf, whom he sometimes called Freedom. He learned that his attentive, adoring bride was fourteen years old.

One thing he had not guessed was the difference that being Pretty Calf's husband would make in his relationship to her mother and brother. He had hoped only to make his position a little safer, but he had not expected to be treated with dignity. Greasy Hand no longer spoke to him at all. When the white man spoke to her, his bride murmured in dismay, explaining at great length that he must never do that. There could be no conversation between a man and his mother-in-law. He could not even mention a word that was part of her name.

Having improved his status so magnificently, he felt no need for hurry in getting away. Now that he had a woman he had as good a chance to be rich as any man. Pretty Calf waited on him; she seldom ran off to play games with other young girls, but took pride in learning from her mother the many women's skills of tanning hides and making clothing and preparing food.

He was no more a horse but a kind of man, a half-Indian, still poor and unskilled but laden with honours, clinging to the buckskin fringes of Crow society.

Escape could wait until he could manage it in comfort, with fit clothing and a good horse, with hunting weapons. Escape could wait until the camp moved near some trading post. He did not plan how he would get home. He dreamed of being there all at once and of telling stories nobody would believe. There was no hurry.

Pretty Calf delighted in educating him. He began to understand tribal arrangements, customs and why things were as they were. They were that way because they had always been so. His young wife giggled when she told him, in his ignorance, things she had always known. But she did not laugh when her brother's wife was taken by another warrior. She explained that solemnly with words and signs.

Yellow Robe belonged to a society called the Big Dogs. The wife-stealer, Cut Neck, belonged to the Foxes. They were fellow tribesmen: they hunted together and fought side by side, but men of one society could take away wives from the other society if they wished, subject to certain limitations.

When Cut Neck rode up to the tepee, laughing and singing, and called to Yellow Robe's wife, 'Come out! Come out!' she did as ordered, looking smug as usual, meek and entirely willing. Thereafter she rode beside him in ceremonial processions and carried his coup stick, while his other wife pretended not to care.

'But why?' the white man demanded of his wife, his Freedom. 'Why did our brother let his woman go? He sits and smokes and does not speak.'

Pretty Calf was shocked at the suggestion. Her brother could not possibly reclaim his woman, she explained. He could not even let her come back if she wanted to—and she probably would want to when Cut Neck tired of her. Yellow Robe could not even admit that his heart was sick. That was the way things were. Deviation meant dishonour.

The woman could have hidden from Cut Neck, she said. She could even have refused to go with him if she had been *ba-wurokee*—a really virtuous woman. But she had been his woman before, for a little while on a berrying expedition, and he had a right to claim her.

There was no sense in it the white man insisted. He glared at his young wife. 'If you go, I will bring you back,' he promised.

She laughed and buried her head against his shoulder. 'I will not have to go,' she said. 'Horse is my first man. There is no hole in my moccasin.'

He stroked her hair and said, '*Ba-wurokee*.'

With great daring, she murmured, '*Hayha*,' and when he did not answer, because he did not know what she meant, she drew away, hurt.

'A woman calls her man that if she thinks he will not leave her. Am I wrong?'

The white man held her closer and lied. 'Pretty Calf is not wrong. Horse will not leave her. Horse will not take another woman, either.' No, he certainly would not. Parting from this one was going to be harder than getting her had been. '*Hayha*,' he murmured. 'Freedom.'

His conscience irked him, but not very much. Pretty Calf could get another man easily enough when he was gone, and a better provider. His hunting skill was improving, but he was still awkward.

There was no hurry about leaving. He was used to most of the Crow ways and could stand the rest. He was becoming prosperous. He owned five horses. His place in the life of the tribe was secure, such as it was. Three or four young women, including the one who had belonged to Yellow Robe, made advances to him. Pretty Calf took pride in the fact that her man was so attractive.

By the time he had what he needed for a secret journey, the grass grew yellow on the plains and the long cold was close. He was enslaved by the girl he called Freedom and, before the winter ended, by the knowledge that she was carrying his child . . .

The Big Dog society held a long ceremony in the spring. The white man strolled with his woman along the creek bank thinking: when I get home I will tell them about the chants and the drumming. Sometime. Sometime.

Pretty Calf would not go to bed when they went back to the tepee.

'Wait and find out about my brother,' she urged. 'Something may happen.'

So far as Horse could figure out, the Big Dogs were having some kind of election. He pampered his wife by staying up with her by the fire. Even the old woman, who was a great one for getting sleep when she was not working, prowled around restlessly.

The white man was yawning by the time the noise of the ceremony died down. When Yellow Robe strode in, garish and heathen in his paint and feathers and furs, the women cried out. There was conversation, too fast for Horse to follow, and the old woman wailed once, but her son silenced her with a gruff command.

When the white man went to sleep he thought his wife was weeping beside him.

The next morning she explained.

'He wears the bearskin belt. Now he can never retreat in battle. He will always be in danger. He will die.'

Maybe he wouldn't, the white man tried to convince her. Pretty Calf recalled that some few men had been honoured by the bearskin belt, vowed to the highest daring, and had not died. If they lived through the summer, then they were free of it.

'My brother wants to die,' she mourned. 'His heart is bitter.'

Yellow Robe lived through half a dozen clashes with small parties of raiders from hostile tribes. His honours were many. He captured horses in any enemy camp, led two successful raids, counted first coup and snatched a gun from the hand of an enemy tribesman. He wore wolf tails on his moccasins and ermine skins on his shirt, and he fringed his leggings with scalps in token of his glory.

When his mother ventured to suggest, as she did many times, 'My son should take a new wife, I need another woman to help me,' he ignored her. He spent much time in prayer, alone in the hills or in conference with a medicine man. He fasted and made vows and kept them. And before he could be free of the heavy honour of the bearskin belt, he went on his last raid.

The warriors were returning from the north just as the white man and two other hunters approached from the south, with buffalo and elk meat dripping from the bloody hides tied on their restive ponies. One of the hunters grunted, and they stopped to watch a rider on the hill north of the tepee circle.

The rider dismounted, held up a blanket and dropped it. He repeated the gesture.

The hunters murmured dismay. 'Two! Two men dead!' They rode fast into the camp, where there was already wailing.

A messenger came down from the war party on the hill. The rest of the party delayed to paint their faces for mourning and for victory. One of the two dead men was Yellow Robe. They had put his body in a cave and walled it in with rocks. The other man died later, and his body was in a tree.

There was blood on the ground before the tepee to which Yellow Robe would return no more. His mother, with her hair chopped short, sat in the doorway, rocking back and forth on her haunches, wailing her heartbreak. She cradled one mutilated hand in the other. She had cut off another finger joint.

Pretty Calf had cut off chunks of her long hair and was crying as she gashed her arms with a knife. The white man tried to take the knife away, but she protested so piteously that he let her do as she wished. He was sickened with the lot of them.

Savages! he thought. Now I will go back! I'll go hunting alone, and I'll keep on going.

But he did not go just yet, because he was the only hunter in the lodge of the two grieving women, one of them old and the other pregnant with his child.

In their mourning they made him a pauper again. Everything that meant comfort, wealth and safety they sacrificed to the spirits because of the death of Yellow Robe. The tepee, made of seventeen fine buffalo hides, the furs that should have kept them warm, the white deerskin dress trimmed with elk teeth that Pretty Calf loved so well, even their tools and Yellow Robe's weapons—everything but his sacred medicine objects—they left there on the prairie, and the whole camp moved away. Two of his best horses were killed as a sacrifice, and the women gave away the rest.

They had no shelter. They would have no tepee of their own for two months at least of mourning, and then the women would have to tan hides to make it. Meanwhile they could live in temporary huts made of willows, covered with skins given them in pity by their friends. They could have lived with relatives, but Yellow Robe's women had no relatives.

The white man had not realized until then how terrible a thing it was for Crow to have no kinfolk. No wonder old Greasy Hand had only stumps for fingers. She had mourned from one year to the next for everyone she had ever loved. She had no-one left but her daughter, Pretty Calf.

Horse was furious at their foolishness. It had been bad enough for him, a captive, to be naked as a horse and poor as a slave, but that was because his captors had stripped him. These women had voluntarily given up everything they needed.

He was too angry at them to sleep in the willow hut. He lay under a sheltering tree. And on the third night of the mourning he made his plans. He had a knife and a bow. He would go after meat, taking two horses. And he would not come back. There were, he realized, many things he was not going to tell when he got back home.

In the willow hut, Pretty Calf cried out. He heard rustling there, and the old woman's querulous voice.

Some twenty hours later his son was born, two months early, in the tepee of a skilled medicine woman. The child was born without breath, and the mother died before the sun went down.

The white man was too shocked to think whether he should mourn, or how he should mourn. The old woman screamed until she was voiceless. Piteously she approached him, bent and trembling, blind with grief. She held out her knife and he took it.

She spread out her hands and shook her head. If she cut off any more finger joints, she could do no more work. She could not afford any more lasting signs of grief.

The white man said, 'All right! All right!' between his teeth.

He hacked his arms with the knife and stood watching the blood run down. It was little enough to do for Pretty Calf, for little Freedom.

Now there is nothing to keep me, he realized. When I get home, I must not let them see the scars.

He looked at Greasy Hand, hideous in her grief-burdened age, and thought: I really am free now! When a wife dies, her husband has no more duty towards her family. Pretty Calf had told him so, long ago, when he wondered why a certain man moved out of one tepee and into another.

The old woman, of course, would be a scavenger. There was one other with the tribe, an ancient crone who had no relatives, toward whom no-one felt any responsibility. She lived on food thrown away by the more fortunate. She slept in shelters that she built with her own knotted hands. She plodded wearily at the end of the procession when the camp moved. When she stumbled, nobody cared. When she died, nobody would miss her.

Tomorrow morning, the white man decided, I will go.

His mother-in-law's sunken mouth quivered. She said one word, questioningly. She said, '*Eero-oshay?*' She said, 'Son?'

Blinking, he remembered. When a wife died, her husband was free. But her mother, who had ignored him with dignity, might if she wished ask him to stay. She invited him by calling him Son, and he accepted by answering Mother.

Greasy Hand stood before him, bowed with years, withered with unceasing labour, loveless and childless, scarred with grief. But with all her burdens she still loved life enough to beg it from him, the only person she had any right to ask. She was stripping herself of all she had left, her pride.

He looked eastward across the prairie. Two thousand miles away was home. The old woman would not live forever. He could afford to wait, for he was young. He could afford to be magnanimous, for he knew he was a man. He gave her the answer. '*Eegya,*' he said. 'Mother.'

He went home three years later. He explained no more than to say, 'I lived with Crows for a while. It was some time before I could leave. They called me Horse.'

He did not find it necessary either to apologize or to boast, because he was the equal of any man on earth.

Uneasy Homecoming *by Will F Jenkins*

Connie began to have the feeling of dread and uneasiness in the taxi but told herself it was not reasonable. She dismissed it decisively when she reached the part of town in which all her friends lived. She could stop and spend the evening with someone until Tom got home, but she didn't. She thrust away the feeling as the taxi rolled out across the neck of land beyond most of the houses. The red, dying sun cast long shadows across the road.

So far, their house was the only one that had been built on the other side of the bay. But she could see plenty of other houses as the taxi drew up before the door. These other houses were across the bay, to be sure, but there was no reason to be upset. She was firm with herself.

The taxi stopped and the last thin sliver of crimson sun went down below the world's edge. Dusk was already here. But everything looked perfectly normal. The house looked neat and hospitable, and it was good to be back. She paid the taxi driver and he obligingly put her suitcases inside the door. The uneasy feeling intensified as he left. But she tried not to heed it.

It continued while she heard the taxi moving away and purring down the road. But it remained essentially the same—a sort of formless restlessness and apprehension—until she went into the kitchen. Then the feeling changed.

She was in the kitchen, with the close smell of a shut-up house about her, when she noticed the change. Her suitcases still lay in the hall where the taxi driver had piled them. The front door was still open to let in fresh air. And quite suddenly she had an urgent conviction that there was something here that she should notice. Something quite inconspicuous. But this sensation was just as absurd as the feeling she'd had in the taxi.

There was a great silence outside the house. This was dusk, and bird and insect noises were growing fainter. There were no neighbours near to make other sounds.

She turned on the refrigerator and it began to make a companionable, humming sound. She turned on the water, and it gushed. But there her queer sensation took a new form. It seemed that every movement produced a noise which advertised her presence, and she felt that there was some reason to be utterly still. And that really was nonsense too.

She glanced into the dining room. She regarded her luggage still piled in the hall near the open front door. Everything looked exactly as everything should look when one returns from a two weeks' holiday and one's husband has been away on business at the same time. Tom would get home about midnight. She had spoken to him on the telephone yesterday. He would positively get back in a few hours. So it would be absurd not to stay here to greet him. The feeling she had, she decided firmly, was simply a normal dislike of being alone. And she would not be silly.

She glanced around the kitchen. Afterwards she remembered that she had looked straight at the back door without seeing what there was to be seen. She went firmly down the hall. Then she went out of doors to look at her flowers.

The garden looked only a little neglected. The west was a fading, already dim glory of red and gold. She could not see too many details, but the garden was fragrant and appealing in the dusk. She saw the garage—locked and empty, of course, since Tom had the car—and felt a minor urge to go over to it. But she did not. Afterwards the memory of that minor urge made her feel faint. But it was only an idea. She dismissed it.

She smelled the comfortable, weary smells of the late summer evening, which would presently give way to the sharper, fresher scents of night. There was the tiny darting shadow of a bat overhead, black against the dark sapphire sky. It was the time when, for a little space, peace seems to enfold all the world. But the nagging uneasiness persisted even out here.

There was a movement by the garage, but it failed to catch her eye. If she had looked—even if she failed to see the movement—she might still have seen the motorcycle. It did not belong here, but it was leaning against the garage wall as if its owner had ridden it here and leaned it confidentially where it would be hidden from anyone looking across the bay. But Connie noticed nothing. She simply felt uneasy.

She found herself going nervously back towards the house. The sunset colours faded, and presently all would be darkness outside. She heard her footsteps on the gravelled walk. Occasional dry leaves brushed against her feet. It seemed to her that she hurried, which was ridiculous. So she forced herself to walk naturally and resisted an impulse to look about.

That was why she failed to notice the pantry window.

She came to the front of the house. Her heels made clicking sounds on the steps. She felt a need to be very quiet, to hide herself.

Yet she had no reason for fear in anything she actually had noticed. She hadn't seen anything odd about the back door or the pantry window, and she hadn't noticed the motorcycle or the movement by the garage. The logical explanation for her feeling of terror was simply that it was dark and she was alone.

She repeated that explanation as she forced herself to enter the dark front doorway.

She wanted to gasp with relief as she felt for the switch and the lights came on. The dark rooms remaining were more terrifying then than the night outside. So she went all over the ground floor, turning on lights, and tried not to think of going upstairs. There was no-one within call and no-one but the taxi driver even knew that she was here. Anything could happen.

But she did not know of anything to cause danger either.

Connie had felt and fought occasional fear before. To bring her nameless frights into the light for scorn, she had talked lightly in the past of the imaginary Things towards which women feel such terror—the Things which nervous women believe are following them; the Things imagined to be hiding in cupboards and behind dark trees in deserted streets. But her past scorn failed to dispel her terror now. She tried to be angry with herself because she was being as silly as the neurotic female who cannot sleep unless she looks under her bed at night. But still, Connie could not drive herself to go upstairs or to look under her own bed right now.

It was an unfortunate omission.

In the lighted living room she had the feeling of someone staring at her from the dark outside. It was unbearable. She went to the telephone, absolutely certain that there was nothing wrong. But if she talked to someone—

She called Mrs Winston. It was not a perfect choice. Mrs Winston was not nearly of Connie's own age, but Connie felt so sorry for the older woman that when she needed comfort she often instinctively called her. Talking to someone else who needed comforting always seemed to make one's own troubles go away.

Mrs Winston's voice was bright and cheery over the phone. 'My dear Connie! How nice it is that you're back with us!'

Connie felt better instantly. She felt herself relaxing, she heard her voice explaining that she'd had a lovely holiday and that Tom was coming back tonight and—

Mrs Winston said anxiously, 'I do hope your house is all right, Connie. Is it? It's been dreadful here! Did you hear?'

'Not a word since I left,' said Connie. 'What's happened?'

She expected to hear about someone having been unkind to Charlie, Mrs Winston's only son. He gave Connie the creeps, but she could feel very sorry for his mother. He had a talent for getting into trouble. There'd been a girl when he was only sixteen, he had been caught stealing in school when there was no excuse for it, and he'd been expelled from college and nowadays wore an apologetic air. Mrs Winston tried to believe that he was simply having a difficult time growing up. But he was already twenty, and at twenty a hulking young man with an apologetic air and a look always thinking of something else—one could sympathize with his mother and still feel uncomfortable about him.

Mrs Winston's voice went on explaining. And the feeling of terror came back upon Connie like a blow.

There had been a series of burglaries in the town. The Hamiltons' house had been ransacked while they were out for an evening's bridge. The Blairs' house was looted while they were away. The Smithsons'. The Tourneys'. And Saddler's shop was robbed, and the burglars seemed to know exactly where Mr Saddler kept his day's receipts and took them and the tray of watches and fountain pens and the cameras. And poor Mr Field—

Mr Field was the ancient cashier at Saddler's. He had interrupted the burglars and they had beaten him horribly, leaving him for dead. He had never regained consciousness, and it was not believed now at the hospital that he ever would.

Connie said from a dry throat, 'I wish you hadn't told me that tonight. I'm all alone. Tom won't be back until midnight.'

'But my dear,' Mrs Winston exclaimed, 'you mustn't. I'll locate Charlie and have him come for you right away! You can spend the evening here and he can take you back when—'

Connie shook her head at the telephone. 'Oh, no! That would be silly!'

She heard her voice refusing, and her mind protested the refusal. But Charlie made her flesh crawl. She could not bear to think of him driving her through the darkness. Baseless terror was bad enough, she thought, without actual aversion besides.

'I'm quite all right!' she insisted. 'Quite! I do hope Mr Field gets better, but I'm all right . . .'

When she hung up the phone she was aware that she was sick. But it was startling to discover that her knees were physically weak when she started to move from the instrument. She could telephone someone else and they would come for her. But Mrs Winston would be offended and take it as an affront. And Connie was still sure that her fear was quite meaningless. It was just a feeling.

She moved aimlessly away from the telephone, found herself at the foot of the stairs. Then she looked up at the dark above and wanted to whimper. But a saving fury came to her. She would not yield to groundless fear. She was in terror of—she called it burglars now, but actually it was of Them, the unknown men women are taught to fear as dangerous.

'Ridiculous!' Connie told herself.

She got a suitcase and started for the stairs. It was deep night now. If she looked out—say, at the garage—she would see nothing. Somewhere there was a dismal cooing. Doves.

She climbed the stairs into darkness. Nothing happened. She pressed a switch and the passage sprang into light. She breathed again. She went into Tom's and her bedroom. There was dust on the dressing table. There was an ashtray. She put down the suitcase and was conscious of bravery because she was angry.

Then she saw cigarette ends on the rug. Scorched places.

Someone had sat here in this bedroom, smoking and indifferently dropping cigarette ends on the rug and crushing them out.

Connie stood with every muscle in her body turned to stone.

A part of Connie's brain directed her eyes again to the bed. Someone had sat on it—only sat—and smoked at leisure. But a corner of the bedspread was twitched aside. What was under the bed? She found herself backing away from it, into a chair which toppled over. The noise made her freeze.

But nothing happened. There was no change in the companionable hum of the refrigerator downstairs. No reaction to the sound of the overturned chair—which seemed incredible. If one of Them—the nameless Things of which she was in terror now—was under the bed, he would come out at the noise.

Presently—her breathing loud in her own ears—Connie bent and looked under the bed. She had to. None of Them was under it. Of course. But there was an object there which was strange.

A very long time later, Connie dragged it out. It was a bag with bulges in it. Her hands shook horribly, but she dumped its contents on the floor. There were cameras. Silver. Sally Hamilton's necklace and rings. There were watches and fountain pens. This must be what the burglars had taken from the Hamiltons' house and the Blairs' and the Smithsons' and the Tourneys'. The cameras and pens and watches came from Saddler's shop, where Mr Field had come upon the burglars and they had beaten him almost to death. The burglars had nearly killed him.

Connie went to the bedroom door. Her knees were water. Her house had been used as the hiding place for the loot of the burglaries that had taken place in her absence. But now if they found out she was back—

Without much rationalization, she could guess why Mr Field had been nearly killed. He must have recognized the burglars. And now they could look across the bay and see that Connie was home. Wouldn't they know instantly that she would soon find their loot? And that she then would telephone for the police . . . ?

Unless they came and stopped her. Quickly.

Shivering, Connie turned out the light in her bedroom. And in the upstairs hall. Downstairs, she turned out the light in the living-room, went quickly to the front door and bolted it. She was leaving it when she thought to fumble her way across the room and make sure that the window was locked. It was. If the lights had been seen across the bay . . . she hastened desperately to turn out the rest. The dining-room. Lights out. The windows were locked. The pantry. It was dark. Whimpering, she was afraid to enter it. She flashed on the light to make sure of the window.

The window was broken. A neat jagged section of glass was missing. It had been cracked and removed so that someone could reach in and unlock it. It was now impossible to lock; anyone could reach in and unfasten it again.

Connie snapped off the light and fled into the kitchen and made that dark. But as the bulb dimmed she realized what she had seen in the very act of snapping the light switch. The back door was not fully closed. Its key was missing. There was mud on the floor where someone had come in—more than once. The burglars must have made casual, constant use of the house.

She stood panting in the blackness. Somewhere outside, frogs croaked. There was a thump, and her heart stood still until she realized that a night-flying insect had bumped against the window.

The refrigerator cut off.

It was coincidence, of course, but it was shocking. The proper thing, the logical thing, was to go to the telephone now. She could not see to dial, but somehow she must.

She felt her way blindly to the instrument. Her fingers on the wall made whispering sounds that guided her and she became aware of the loud pounding sound her heart made.

Just as she reached the telephone there was a faint noise which might have been a footstep in the garden.

She waited, filled with such fear that her body did not seem to exist and she had no physical sensation at all.

But a part of her brain saw with infinite despair that if the burglars had been near the house at sunset, intending to enter it as soon as darkness fell, they would have seen the taxi deliver her. They would have known that sooner or later she would discover proof of their presence. And what she had just done told them of her discovery! The light in the bedroom where their loot was hidden turned out . . . Every other light turned out. They would know she had darkened the house to hide in it, to use the telephone.

There was a soft sound at the back door. It squeaked.

Connie stood rigid. The clicking of the dial would tell everything. She could not conceivably summon help.

There was the soft whisper of a foot on the kitchen linoleum. Connie's hands closed convulsively. The one thought that came to her now was that she must breathe quietly.

There was a grey glow somewhere. The figure in the kitchen was throwing a torch beam on the floor. Then it halted, waiting. He knew that she was hiding somewhere in the house.

He went almost soundlessly into the living-room. She saw the glow of the light there. Back into the kitchen. She heard him moving quietly—listening—towards the door through which she had come only a few seconds before to use the telephone.

He came through that door, within three feet of her. But when he was fully through the doorway she was behind him. Again he flashed the light downwards. But he did not think to look behind him. By just so much she was saved for the moment.

In the greyish light reflected from the floor she recognized him.

He went into the dining-room. He moved very quietly, but he bumped ever so slightly against a chair. The noise made her want to shriek. He was hunting her, and he knew that she was in the house and he had to kill her. He had to get his loot and get away, and she must not be able to tell anything about him.

He was back in the kitchen again. He stood there, listening, and Connie was aware of a new and added emotion which came of her recognition of him. She felt that she would lie down at any instant and scream—because she knew him!

He came towards the door again, but he went up the stairs. They creaked under his weight. He must have reasoned cunningly that she would want to hide, because she was afraid. So he would go into the bedroom and look under the bed . . .

Connie slipped her feet out of her slippers. He had not reached the top of the stairs before she stood in her stockinged feet in the blackness below.

The front door was impossible. She would have to unlock it, make a noise. But he had not closed the back door behind him.

She crept out of it, with a passionate care that almost vanished when she was in the blessed night. There were stars. She remembered that she must not step on the gravel on which her feet might make a noise, so she stepped on the grass. And she fled.

There were sounds inside the house. He was opening cupboards, deliberately making sounds to fill her with panic as he hunted her down. He hadn't guessed yet that she was outside.

There were shrubs by the garage, so she slowed her flight to avoid them. And then she came upon the motorcycle. She smelled it, oil and petrol and rubber. It was useless to her. She had no idea how to operate it. But suddenly a wild escape occurred to her—the motorcycle wasn't entirely useless.

Connie fumbled with the machine. She turned a little tap. The smell of petrol grew strong. There was a crash inside the house. But outside the night was full of stars, and the air was cool and sweet—except that the smell of petrol was growing stronger in it.

Connie had a box of matches in her pocket. Quickly she got it out, and in one motion struck a match and dropped it and ran away into the darkness, with the strange feel of grass under her feet.

The petrol blazed fiercely. She hid herself in the shadows and watched, sobs trying to form in her throat. The fire would be seen across the bay. It would plainly be at Connie's house. People would come quickly—a lot of them. And fire engines.

As the flames grew higher, she saw the figure plunge from the house, run furiously towards the fire, try to flail it out. But it was impossible.

And he knew it. Even his twisted mind would tell him that nothing could hide his identity now. The motorcycle would be identification enough, and there was the loot in the house.

Connie found herself weeping. It was partly relief. But it

was also the unnerving realization that the fears she'd had about Them, the men who prey on others, were not entirely groundless.

The headlights of cars began to focus towards the house, along the road from the mainland. The bells of fire engines started tolling and grew louder. And in the leaping flames surrounding the motorcycle, a hulking, desperate figure threw futile handfuls of earth upon the machine. Was he, Connie wondered, trying to create the hopeless pretence that he was the first to help?

Even so, she was quite safe now, Connie knew. She began to cry in reaction from her terror. But, also, she wept heartbrokenly for poor Mrs Winston. She, Connie, could have been murdered. She could have been the victim of one of those twisted men who prey on their fellow beings. But she wept for Mrs Winston.

She, Connie, would not now be one of the women They had killed. But Mrs Winston was the mother of one of Them.

Natuk *by George Bruce*

I was stationed, at one period of my service with the Mounted Police, in the far north of Canada, on the Porcupine River, some fifty miles north of Rat Lake. Though well on the cool side of the Arctic Circle, we were just then having our short hot summer. The day temperature often rose to eighty degrees, and in the evenings there seemed to be more mosquitoes than fresh air. My cabin stood by a small lake from which a stream ran down to the river, among low hills covered with spruce forest.

I spent many hours roaming through that forest, or sitting still, watching the wild life that filled it. Among bracken and brambles, fallen trees and branches, it was easy to find a hiding place from which one could see all round.

There was plenty to see if a man stayed quiet and kept his eyes open: birds of many sorts, foxes, martens, squirrels, mink, the friendly little chipmunks, perhaps a deer, perhaps a she-wolf with a small cub, a lumbering bear in search of food, or a porcupine stripping the rough outer bark from a sapling spruce, to feed on the succulent inner skin.

One day I had been for a long walk through the woods and was on my way back when I came upon a wolverine trap. It had been sprung, and in it, lying dead, was a beautiful husky bitch. She must have run away from some Indian camp, the call of her wolf ancestors in her blood, and taken to the woods.

The trap had been set for wolves or wolverines, pestilent brutes both, and it was clearly right that I should set it again. I forced down the spring till I could open the powerful spiked jaws, and was pulling out the dead husky when I heard a whimper. Out from under the body crawled a little pup, only a few weeks old. I tucked him into the breast of my coat and reset the trap, after which I skinned the husky, thinking that her pelt would make a good rug for my cabin, and then started for home.

My dogs were tied up, but when I put the pup down and began to open the cabin door they scented him, and a savage growl arose that told of their smelling possible food. The pup sensed danger and huddled close to my feet as I entered the cabin.

I fed him on condensed milk till he was old enough to eat solid food, and at night he would curl up in my bunk with me. Before long he would follow me everywhere unless I had to go out for the day, when he would settle down on the rug beside my bed, the rug I had made out of his mother's skin. Evidently he found some friendly influence in it, for while I was away he would lie there quite happily and never move.

After the first week I introduced him formally to the sledge dogs. They sniffed him over, each in turn, and then accepted him as a regular member of the household. Soon he would take all manner of liberties with them, usually borne with amused tolerance, but if he went too far—if, for example, he tugged too vigorously with his sharp little teeth at a big dog's ear—a growl and a warning snap of teeth would follow. The pup would flee in any direction and lie low till the atmosphere cleared.

My team leader especially became very attached to the youngster. When I took the sledge out I would put the pup on top of the load, and the team leader soon recognized this as part of the regular routine. Before starting he would look round to see that the pup was on the load. If he was not, no shouts or whip-cracks would induce the leader to start till the pup was duly installed.

From the first I decided that he was not to be a sledge dog, but my personal companion; and a splendid companion he proved. He came with me on all my rambles through the woods, and if I was looking for meat he would put up rabbits for me to shoot. I soon trained him not to chase them, and as his intelligence developed I taught him many things. I would leave some article on the doorstep and send him back to fetch it, till he would do so from a long distance. Later I would give him something, a glove or mitten, sending him home to leave it on the mat and return.

Perhaps because he was never treated as harshly as one has to treat sledge dogs, he showed a sensitive nature such as I have known in no other husky. I never once had to beat him; a tap of my fingers on his nose was the utmost correction he needed, and he would look up with a pathetic expression as much as to say, 'What have I done wrong?' As a watchdog he was unsurpassed. No stranger could approach the cabin unless I introduced him, when the dog would sniff him all over with a low throaty growl, and would never fail to know him if he came again.

By the time he had grown to his full size, a magnificent dog, we were inseparable companions. He would hardly let me out of his sight; wherever I went he followed close at my heels. I called him 'Natuk', which in the West Eskimo language means 'shadow'. We lived alone, far from any human society, and our comradeship grew closer and closer as time went on, until I used to feel that he knew exactly what I was thinking about.

A handsome animal was Natuk, about thirty inches at the shoulder and weighing close on nine stone. His colour was that of a sable collie, but a few shades lighter, with dark tips to the long hair, especially on his flanks, while his broad chest was almost white. Probably his sire was a timber-wolf for he had the true wolf head with sharp prick-ears, though a white blaze on his face suggested a strain of Newfoundland in his dam, which may have accounted for his weight and strength. His bushy tail was carried in proper husky style, close-curled over his back.

My position in the Mounted Police was officially that of doctor, but in that sparsely-populated region the calls for medical or surgical help were few, and unofficially I did a good deal of regular police work, especially in the matter of keeping an eye on any strangers who might drift into the country, and finding out all about them. Some fifty miles away lived a friend of mine, a Dogrib Indian, whom I found very useful in getting me information of this kind, information which I passed on to the proper quarter.

Early in October a rumour reached me of two newcomers to the district who did not sound desirable visitors. I decided to look up my Indian friend and see what he could tell me about them. The first snow had already fallen, and as usual, before the weather grows really cold, it was soft and yielding.

Snow of that kind makes bad travelling for a dog sledge, and fifty miles being a short journey as we reckon things in the North, I planned to do it on foot, pulling a light toboggan with the few things I needed—rifle, blankets, food, and a small tent.

Natuk, of course, would come with me, and my Indian chore-boy would look after the sledge dogs till my return.

About twenty-five miles out, halfway to my destination, was the cabin of my nearest neighbour, a Swedish trapper and a good friend of mine. Ole Oleson was a man with more education than the average trapper, and a better philosophy of life.

In the spring, when he took his winter's harvest of furs to the trading-post, instead of spending the proceeds in a riotous orgy, he would bank most of the money and come back to the North to earn more. He was now a well-to-do man. His cabin was comfortable beyond the ordinary standard; he was intelligent and a good talker, and I always enjoyed an evening with him.

Starting early, Natuk and I reached Ole's cabin late in the afternoon. We had a hearty welcome from the trapper, and spent a pleasant evening. Next morning after breakfast I began to pack my gear on the toboggan, when Ole begged me not to go.

'There's a blizzard coming,' he said. 'Stop here today, and you can go when it has blown over.'

Ole was an experienced backwoodsman, but so was I, having been born and brought up in that country. I looked at the sky.

'You're wrong, Ole,' I said.

'I'm not,' said he. 'I know it's coming. I can smell it.'

I did not believe him, and I said so. I was anxious to push on, as I felt it was important to see the Indian and get him onto those two strangers before they could start any funny business. But Ole insisted, and the end of it was that we lit our pipes and sat talking and smoking till well after midday. Then I decided that I could delay no longer, so I finished packing the toboggan and said, 'Well, Ole, if I *do* get into a jam, I'll send Natuk back to you and he'll guide you to wherever I happen to be.'

Natuk and I set out, taking a trail that led through the upper hills where the spruce forest was thin and open. The sun went down about three o'clock, and with its setting a wind sprang up, growing rapidly stronger. I began to think that Ole might be right about the blizzard, and turned downhill towards the thick spruce in the valley, which would give some shelter.

I was going as fast as I could when suddenly the ground gave way under my feet, and I dropped into space. Throwing out my hands instinctively to save myself, I let go the rope, and the toboggan skidded away among the trees.

In a moment I realized what had happened. I had fallen into an Indian bear-trap, scores of which were to be found in these hills. A wide pit is dug, about eight feet deep, one or more pointed stakes fixed in the bottom, and the top crossed by stretchers of young saplings over which is laid a cover of brushwood. The snow had hidden the trap effectively, and I had walked straight into it.

Not having the weight or bulk of a bear, I had not gone to the bottom. I was caught round the waist by a mass of jagged sticks, the upper part of my body free, but on kicking about to try for some foothold I found that the pit was full of brambles and dead twigs that had fallen through the cover. This meant that the trap was an old one, perhaps several years old.

That set me thinking. Probably the stretchers covering the trap were pretty rotten. If I struggled too violently the whole thing might collapse and land me at the bottom of the pit, where the pointed hardwood stakes might still be sound enough and sharp enough to impale me. Even if they were not, it would be impossible to climb out, and I should starve to death miserably in that tangle of dead sticks and brambles.

Cautiously I tried to work my way out of the mass of spiky branches that gripped me, but in vain. I had no foothold to give me a leg up, and my efforts only resulted in my sinking a few inches lower. The wind was blowing a gale now, and I could hear dead trees falling far and near.

Suddenly a sharp crack sounded close by. A dead spruce, split by the frost of some previous winter, broke off, the whole top of one half falling across the bear-trap and pinning me down. I was not much hurt, but only my right arm remained free; my left arm and my body were held as in a vice among the network of broken boughs and debris.

All this time Natuk had been jumping round me, scratching in the snow, trying to dig me out, and pulling at sticks with his teeth. Several times he broke through the top crust, but having four legs he was able to scramble out. Now that I was helplessly pinioned, it flashed through my mind that he might really be able to assist me. I had said jokingly to Ole that if I got into a jam I would send Natuk to fetch him. That joke could be turned into reality if Natuk was as clever as I believed him to be.

When I came in from a journey I would often get him to pull off my big moose-hide mittens, and now I called him, holding out my free right hand till he caught the end of the mitten in his teeth. As he pulled it off I said, 'Take it back and get help, Natuk!' waving my hand in the direction of Ole's cabin. Natuk looked at me as if trying to grasp what I was saying; then, as I repeated the order and pointed to the way, he seemed to catch the idea. With one snap he gripped the mitten firmly in his mouth and set off at a loping wolf-canter on the line that I had given him.

There I was, left all alone, with plenty of time to think things over. I began to calculate when I might expect help to come. We had covered about ten miles when I turned off the trail.

With the wild animal's instinct for short-cuts, Natuk should bring that down to seven miles at the most, and he could do that in an hour. It should not take Ole more than an hour and a half to harness up his dog-team and come out. So in two hours and a half, three hours at the most, I might expect to be released.

The wind dropped as quickly as it had risen, and in an hour's time the air was again perfectly still. Not a sound of any kind in the woods, only the dead silence of an Arctic winter's night. Though there was no moon it was by no means dark, as the brilliance of the stars in that clear air, refracted from the snow, gives light enough to see things fairly well at a short distance.

In my constrained position, half lying with my feet unsupported, I grew very stiff and cold, especially my right arm. When the tree fell I had thrown it up to guard my head, with the result that a forked branch had trapped it so that I could not bring my hand lower than my shoulder.

Now that the heavy moose-hide mitten was gone, I had no protection for that hand but the woollen inner mitten. It was lucky for me that the wind had dropped, or I should have been frost-bitten. Round me was a cage of bare branches; in front of me the long split trunk of the spruce.

Slowly the time crawled on, while I tried to picture my dog racing through the woods to the trapper's cabin; the hurried harnessing of the dog-team, and the Swede dashing along the trail; Natuk, ahead of the team, going all out to bring help to his master and friend.

Then through the profound silence of the winter woods rang a blood-freezing cry, the howl of a lone wolf.

There is a difference between the howl of a wolf that leads a pack, on first scenting his quarry, and that of a solitary beast, the ex-leader of a pack, driven from his position by a younger and stronger rival. The difference is not to be described in words, but the lone wolf's howl has an indefinable quality which a trained ear cannot mistake, an aggressive and defiant note, as if voicing the bitterness that rankles in the heart of the deposed leader.

That sense of defeat, joined to the craft and cunning which years of leadership have given him, makes the lone wolf the most dangerous beast in all the North.

I could hear that cry now, its low cadence gradually working up to the full-throated howl, then dying away. A long pause, ten minutes at least, and it came again, this time nearer and louder. Once more it sounded, nearer still, and then the deep silence of the night. I listened with every nerve strung. Was it my scent that the hunter had winded, or that of some night-roaming animal?

Near the butt of the fallen spruce I suddenly saw two points of green light. They moved forward, and behind them I could just make out a ghostly form creeping along the tree-trunk. I shouted, and the brute backed; but soon he crept forward again.

Again I shouted, and again, and each time he drew back. Once or twice he disappeared for a short time, but returned. I kept on shouting till my voice dropped to a hoarse croak. The wolf grew bolder, and came on slowly till he was about ten feet away.

In spite of the peril of my position I could not help feeling the grim humour of it. Here was I, a grown man in full health and strength, at the mercy of a beast not half my size. Born and reared in these northern forests, trained from childhood in all the woodcraft and hunting lore of the Indians, I felt that the rawest tenderfoot could not have got himself into a worse mess.

My revolver, a Colt's .45, capable of killing six wolves in ten seconds, hung from my belt fully loaded. But I could not get either hand down to draw it, and the wolf was master of the situation. The thing was just absurd.

Absurd or not, however, I must do what I could while any hope remained. Indian hunters had often told me that a wolf will never attack so long as a man keeps up some rhythmic motion. I began to wave my right hand in a measured swing from side to side, and I could see the wolf's head and eyes following the movement. He stood there half crouched, a lean, hungry-looking brute, saliva dripping from his jaws, and those baleful green eyes glowing dimly in the starlight; but he came no nearer.

I was numb with cold, and my arm grew so weary with the steady movement that I began to wonder how long I could keep it up. The chill of utter exhaustion was creeping over me. Soon I should be unable to swing my hand any more, and then . . .

Three shots rang out—distant, but clear in the still night air. Ole was firing to signal his coming. A rush of hope surged through me, lending a momentary spasm of energy to my weary arm. But the sound of those shots seemed to rouse the wolf from his inaction, as if he felt that his time was short and that he must get to work. With fangs bared he began to creep nearer. My strength was almost gone; another moment and those fangs would be at my throat.

A heavy body hurtled through the air. Natuk, his teeth buried in the wolf's shoulder, flung him off the tree, and the two were locked in a fierce grapple in the hollow of the bear-trap. The snow flew in showers as the fight maddened to fury.

Both fought silently after the manner of wolves, not a sound but the snap and slash of teeth and the dull rip of skin and flesh. If ever I prayed in my life, I prayed then that my dog might win.

The duel went on, fierce and deadly, both combatants fighting to kill. If Natuk was a shade the heavier, the wolf was an experienced brute that had fought his way to the head of the pack and kept his position for years by dint of ferocity and fangs. For a time I could not tell which was getting the better of it.

At length the wolf bounded out of the hollow on to the level ground. Natuk leaped after him, and the death-worry began again. I saw Natuk grip the wolf by the side of the neck, and throw him clean over his back. Then I must have fainted, for I knew no more till I heard the crack of a pistol—Ole finishing off the wolf.

It seemed ages before Ole dragged me clear of the bear-trap. I was too spent to give him any help, and it needed all his great strength to pull me out. My first thought was to look at Natuk.

He lay on the blood-soaked snow, hideously mauled, a mass of wounds. Both shoulders were torn to the bone, one ear was slashed off, his flank ripped open to the ribs, and the entrails sagging out. But his eyes spoke to me dumbly, and he tried to lick my hand.

We of the North have not much use for sentiment. Life is too hard and death too near at all times to encourage any soft-hearted emotions, and my upbringing among the Indians had case-hardened my feelings since childhood.

But the sight of my friend and comrade lying there in such agony brought me nearer to a breakdown than ever before or since. Yet the wolf was in a worse state, and it can hardly have needed Ole's bullet to give him the *coup de grâce*.

Natuk was dying, but he had won the battle.

I knew too much of wounds to have any hope. The only kindness I could show Natuk was to put him out of his pain. I drew my revolver, but the look in the dog's eyes was too much for me. 'Ole,' I said, 'I'll leave it to you to do him the good turn.'

Sick at heart, I crept away among the bushes, pulling my coat over my head, till through the heavy fur I heard a muffled report and knew that all was over. We put Natuk on the sledge, and next day I buried him in a clearing near the trapper's cabin, where the sun would shine upon his grave. At its head I placed a heavy wooden slab, and on it cut three words deeply with my knife—

NATUK MY SHADOW

Dip in the Pool *by Roald Dahl*

On the morning of the third day, the sea calmed. Even the most delicate passengers—those who had not been seen around the ship since sailing time—emerged from their cabins and crept up onto the sun deck, where the deck steward gave them chairs and tucked rugs around their legs and left them lying in rows, their faces upturned to the pale, almost heatless January sun.

It had been moderately rough the first two days, and this sudden calm and the sense of comfort that it brought created a more genial atmosphere over the whole ship. By the time evening came, the passengers, with twelve hours of good weather behind them, were beginning to feel confident, and at eight o'clock that night the main dining-room was filled with people eating and drinking with the assured, complacent air of seasoned sailors.

The meal was not half over when the passengers became aware, by a slight friction between their bodies and the seats of their chairs, that the big ship had actually started rolling again. It was very gentle at first, just a slow, lazy leaning to one side, then to the other, but it was enough to cause a subtle, immediate change of mood over the whole room. A few of the passengers glanced up from their food, hesitating, waiting, almost listening for the next roll, smiling nervously, little secret glimmers of apprehension in their eyes. Some were completely unruffled, some were openly smug, a number of the smug ones making jokes about food and weather in order to torture the few who were beginning to suffer. The movement of the ship then became rapidly more and more violent, and only five or six minutes after the first roll had been noticed, she was swinging heavily from side to side, the passengers bracing themselves in their chairs, leaning against the pull, as in a car cornering.

At last the really bad roll came, and Mr William Botibol, sitting at the purser's table, saw his plate of poached turbot with hollandaise sauce sliding suddenly away from under his fork. There was a flutter of excitement, everyone reaching for plates and wineglasses. Mrs Renshaw, seated at the purser's right, gave a little scream and clutched that gentleman's arm.

'Going to be a dirty night,' the purser said, looking at Mrs Renshaw. 'I think it's blowing up for a very dirty night.' There was just the faintest suggestion of relish in the way he said it.

A steward came hurrying up and sprinkled water on the tablecloth between the plates. The excitement subsided. Most of the passengers continued with their meal. A small number, including Mrs Renshaw, got carefully to their feet and threaded their ways with a kind of concealed haste between the tables and through the doorway.

'Well,' the purser said, 'there she goes.' He glanced around with approval at the remainder of his flock, who were sitting quiet, looking complacent, their faces reflecting openly that extraordinary pride that travellers seem to take in being recognized as 'good sailors'.

When the eating was finished and the coffee had been served, Mr Botibol, who had been unusually grave and thoughtful since the rolling started, suddenly stood up and carried his cup of coffee around to Mrs Renshaw's vacant place, next to the purser. He seated himself in her chair, then immediately leaned over and began to whisper urgently in the purser's ear. 'Excuse me,' he said, 'but could you tell me something please?'

The purser, small and fat and red, bent forward to listen. 'What's the trouble, Mr Botibol?'

'What I want to know is this.' The man's face was anxious and the purser was watching it. 'What I want to know is will the captain already have made his estimate on the day's run—you know, for the auction pool? I mean before it began to get rough like this?'

The purser, who had prepared himself to receive a personal confidence, smiled and leaned back in his seat to relax his full belly. 'I should say so—yes,' he answered. He did not bother to whisper his reply, although automatically he lowered his voice, as one does when answering a whisperer.

'About how long ago do you think he did it?'

'Some time this afternoon. He usually does it in the afternoon.'

'About what time?'

'Oh, I don't know. Around four o'clock I should guess.'

'Now tell me another thing. How does the captain decide which number it shall be? Does he take a lot of trouble over that?'

The purser looked at the anxious frowning face of Mr Botibol and he smiled, knowing quite well what the man was driving at. 'Well, you see, the captain has a little conference with the navigating officer, and they study the weather and a lot of other things, and then they make their estimate.'

Mr Botibol nodded, pondering this answer for a moment. Then he said, 'Do you think the captain knew there was bad weather coming today?'

'I couldn't tell you,' the purser replied. He was looking into the small black eyes of the other man, seeing the two single little sparks of excitement dancing in their centres. 'I really couldn't tell you, Mr Botibol. I wouldn't know.'

'If this gets any worse it might be worth buying some of the low numbers. What do you think?' The whispering was more urgent, more anxious now.

'Perhaps it will,' the purser said. 'I doubt the old man allowed for a really rough night. It was pretty calm this afternoon when he made his estimate.'

The others at the table had become silent and were trying to hear, watching the purser with that intent, half-cocked, listening look that you can see also at the race track when they are trying to overhear a trainer talking about his chance: the slightly open lips, the upstretched eyebrows, the head forward and cocked a little to one side—that desperately straining, half-hypnotized, listening look that comes to all of them when they are hearing something straight from the horse's mouth.

'Now supposing *you* were allowed to buy a number, which one would *you* choose today?' Mr Botibol whispered.

'I don't know what the range is yet,' the purser patiently answered. 'They don't announce the range till the auction starts after dinner. And I'm really not very good at it anyway. I'm only the purser, you know.'

At that point Mr Botibol stood up. 'Excuse me, all,' he said, and he walked carefully away over the swaying floor between the other tables, and twice he had to catch hold of the back of a chair to steady himself against the ship's roll.

'The sun deck, please,' he said to the elevator man.

The wind caught him full in the face as he stepped out onto the open deck. He staggered and grabbed hold of the rail and held on tight with both hands, and he stood there looking out over the darkening sea where the great waves were welling up high, and white horses were riding against the wind with plumes of spray behind them as they went.

'Pretty bad out there, wasn't it, sir?' the elevator man said on the way down.

Mr Botibol was combing his hair back into place with a small red comb. 'Do you think we've slackened speed at all on account of the weather?' he asked.

'Oh my word yes, sir. We slacked off considerable since this started. You got to slacken off speed in weather like this or you'll be throwing passengers all over the ship.'

Down in the smoking-room people were already gathering for the auction. They were grouping themselves politely around the various tables, the men a little stiff in their dinner jackets, a little pink and overshaved and stiff beside their cool, white-armed women. Mr Botibol took a chair close to the auctioneer's table. He crossed his legs, folded his arms, and settled himself in his seat with the rather desperate air of a man who has made a tremendous decision and refuses to be frightened.

The pool, he was telling himself, would probably be around seven thousand dollars. That was almost exactly what it had been the last two days, with the numbers selling for between three and four hundred apiece. Being a British ship they did it in pounds, but he liked to do his thinking in his own currency. Seven thousand dollars was plenty of money. My goodness yes! And what he would do, he would get them to pay him in hundred-dollar bills and he would take it ashore in the inside pocket of his jacket. No problem there. And right away, yes right away, he would buy a Lincoln convertible. He would pick it up on the way from the ship and drive it home just for the pleasure of seeing Ethel's face when she came out of the front door and looked at it. Wouldn't that really be something, to see Ethel's face when he glided up to the door in a brand-new pale-green Lincoln convertible! Hello Ethel honey, he would say, speaking very casually. I just thought I'd get you a little present. I saw it in the window as I went by, so I thought of you and how you were always wanting one. You like it, honey? he would say. You like the colour? and then he would watch her face.

The auctioneer was standing up behind his table now. 'Ladies and gentlemen!' he shouted. 'The captain has estimated the day's run, ending at midday tomorrow, at five hundred and fifteen miles. As usual we will take the ten numbers on either side of it to make up the range. That makes it five hundred and five to five hundred and twenty-five. And of course for those who think the true figure will be still farther away, there'll be "low field" and "high field" sold separately as well. Now, we'll draw the first number out of the hat . . . here we are . . . five hundred and twelve . . . what am I bid for number five hundred and twelve?'

The room became quiet. The people sat still in their chairs, all eyes watching the auctioneer. There was a certain tension in the air, and as the bids got higher, the tension grew. This wasn't a game or a joke: you could be sure of that by the way that one man would look across at another who had raised his bid—smiling perhaps, but only the lips smiling, the eyes bright and absolutely cold.

Number five hundred and twelve was knocked down for one hundred and ten pounds. The next three or four numbers fetched roughly the same amount.

The ship was rolling heavily, and each time she went over, the wooden panelling on the walls creaked as if it were going to split. The passengers held on to the arms of their chairs, concentrating upon the auction.

'Low field!' the auctioneer called out. 'The next number is low field.'

Mr Botibol sat up very straight and tense. He would wait, he had decided, until the others had finished bidding, then he would jump in and make the last bid. He had figured that there must be at least five hundred dollars in his account at the bank at home, probably nearer six. That was about two hundred pounds—over two hundred. This ticket wouldn't fetch more than that.

'As you all know,' the auctioneer was saying, 'low field covers every number *below* the smallest number in the range, in this case every number below five hundred and five. So if you think this ship is going to cover less than five hundred and five miles in the twenty-four hours ending at noon tomorrow, you'd better get in and buy this number. So what am I bid?'

It went clear up to one hundred and thirty pounds. Others besides Mr Botibol seemed to have noticed that the weather was rough. One hundred and forty . . . fifty . . . There it stopped. The auctioneer raised his hammer.

'Going at one hundred and fifty . . .'

'Sixty!' Mr Botibol called, and every face in the room turned and looked at him.

'Seventy!'

'Eighty!' Mr Botibol called.

'Ninety!'

'Two hundred!' Mr Botibol called. He wasn't stopping now—not for anyone.

There was a pause.

'Any advance on two hundred pounds?'

Sit still, he told himself. Sit absolutely still and don't look up. It's unlucky to look up. Hold your breath. No-one's going to bid you up so long as you hold your breath.

'Going for two hundred pounds . . .' The auctioneer had a pink bald head and there were little beads of sweat sparkling on top of it. 'Going . . .' Mr Botibol held his breath. '. . . Going . . . Gone!' The man banged the hammer on the table. Mr Botibol wrote out a cheque and handed it to the auctioneer's assistant, then he settled back in his chair to wait for the finish. He did not want to go to bed before he knew how much there was in the pool.

They added it up after the last number had been sold and it came to twenty-one hundred-odd pounds. That was around six thousand dollars. Ninety per cent to go to the winner, ten per cent to seamen's charities. Ninety per cent of six thousand was five thousand four hundred. Well—that was enough. He could buy the Lincoln convertible and there would be something left over, too. With this gratifying thought he went off, happy and excited, to his cabin.

When Mr Botibol awoke the next morning he lay quite still

for several minutes with his eyes shut, listening for the sound of the gale, waiting for the roll of the ship. There was no sound of any gale and the ship was not rolling. He jumped up and peered out of the porthole. The sea was smooth as glass, the great ship was moving through it fast, obviously making up for time lost during the night. Mr Botibol turned away and sat slowly down on the edge of his bunk. A fine electricity of fear was beginning to prickle under the skin of his stomach. He hadn't a hope now. One of the higher numbers was certain to win it after this.

'Oh my God,' he said aloud. 'What shall I do?'

What, for example, would Ethel say? It was simply not possible to tell her that he had spent almost all of their two years' savings on a ticket in the ship's pool. Nor was it possible to keep the matter secret. To do that he would have to tell her to stop drawing cheques. And what about the monthly instalments on the television set and the *Encyclopaedia Britannica*? Already he could see the anger and contempt in the woman's eyes, the blue becoming grey and the eyes themselves narrowing as they always did when there was anger in them.

'Oh my God. What *shall* I do?'

There was no point in pretending that he had the slightest chance now—not unless the ship started to go backwards. They'd have to put her in reverse and go full speed astern and keep right on going if he was to have any chance of winning it now. Well, maybe he should ask the captain to do just that. Offer him ten per cent of the profits. Offer him more if he wanted it. Mr Botibol started to giggle. Then very suddenly he stopped, his eyes and mouth both opening wide in a kind of shocked surprise. For it was at this moment that the idea came. It hit him hard and quick, and he jumped up from his bed, terribly excited, ran over to the porthole and looked out again. Well, he thought, why not? Why ever not? The sea was calm and he wouldn't have any trouble keeping afloat until they picked him up. He had a vague feeling that someone had done this thing before, but that didn't prevent him from doing it again. The ship would have to stop and lower a boat, and the boat would have to go back maybe half a mile to get him, and then it would have to return to the ship and be hoisted back on board. It would take at least an hour, the whole thing.

An hour was about thirty miles. It would knock thirty miles off the day's run. That would do it. 'Low field' would be sure to win it then. Just so long as he made certain someone saw him falling over; but that would be simple to arrange. And he'd better wear light clothes, something easy to swim in. Sports clothes, that was it. He would dress as though he were going up to play some deck tennis—just a shirt and a pair of shorts and tennis-shoes. And leave his watch behind. What was the time? Nine-fifteen. The sooner the better, then. Do it now and get it over with. Have to do it soon, because the time limit was midday.

Mr Botibol was both frightened and excited when he stepped out onto the sun deck in his sports clothes. His small body was wide at the hips, tapering upward to extremely narrow, sloping shoulders, so that it resembled, in shape at any rate, a bollard. His white, skinny legs were covered with black hairs, and he came cautiously out on deck, treading softly in his tennis shoes. Nervously he looked around him. There was only one other person in sight, an elderly woman with very thick ankles and immense buttocks who was leaning over the rail staring at the sea. She was wearing a coat of Persian lamb and the collar was turned up so Mr Botibol couldn't see her face.

He stood still, examining her carefully from a distance. Yes, he told himself, she would probably do. She would probably give the alarm just as quickly as anyone else. But wait one minute, take your time, William Botibol, take your time. Remember what you told yourself a few minutes ago in the cabin when you were changing? You remember that?

The thought of leaping off a ship into the ocean a thousand miles from the nearest land had made Mr Botibol—a cautious man at the best of times—unusually advertent. He was by no means satisfied yet that this woman he saw before him was *absolutely certain* to give the alarm when he made his jump. In his opinion there were two possible reasons why she might fail him. Firstly, she might be deaf and blind. It was not very probable, but on the other hand it *might* be so, and why take a chance? All he had to do was check it by talking to her for a moment beforehand. Secondly—and this will demonstrate how suspicious the mind of a man can become when it is working through self-preservation and fear—secondly, it had occurred to him that the woman might herself be the owner of one of the high numbers in the pool and, as such, would have a sound financial reason for not wishing to stop the ship. Mr Botibol recalled that people had killed their fellows for far less than six thousand dollars. It was happening every day in the newspapers. So why take a chance on that either? Check on it first. Be sure of your facts. Find out about it by a little polite conversation. Then provided that the woman appeared also to be a pleasant, kindly human being, the thing was a cinch and he could leap overboard with a light heart.

Mr Botibol advanced casually toward the woman and took up a position beside her, leaning on the rail. 'Hullo,' he said pleasantly.

She turned and smiled at him, a surprisingly lovely, almost a beautiful smile, although the face itself was very plain. 'Hullo,' she answered him.

Check, Mr Botibol told himself, on the first question. She is neither blind nor deaf. 'Tell me,' he said, coming straight to the point, 'what did you think of the auction last night?'

'Auction?' she asked, frowning. 'Auction? What auction?'

'You know, that silly old thing they have in the lounge after dinner, selling numbers on the ship's daily run. I just wondered what you thought about it.'

She shook her head, and again she smiled, a sweet and pleasant smile that had in it perhaps the trace of an apology. 'I'm very lazy,' she said. 'I always go to bed early. I have my dinner in bed. It's so restful to have dinner in bed.'

Mr Botibol smiled back at her and began to edge away. 'Got to go and get my exercise now,' he said. 'Never miss my exercise in the morning. It was nice seeing you. Very nice seeing you . . .' He retreated about ten paces, and the woman let him go without looking around.

Everything was now in order. The sea was calm, he was lightly dressed for swimming, there were almost certainly no man-eating sharks in this part of the Atlantic, and there was this pleasant, kindly old woman to give the alarm. It was a question now only of whether the ship would be delayed long enough to swing the balance in his favour. Almost certainly it would. In any event, he could do a little to help in that direction himself. He could make a few difficulties about getting hauled up into the lifeboat. Swim around a bit, back away from them surreptitiously as they tried to come up close to fish him out. Every minute, every second gained would help him win. He began to move forward again to the rail, but now a new fear assailed him. Would he get caught in the propeller? He had heard about that happening to persons falling off the sides of big ships. But then, he wasn't going to fall, he was going to jump, and that was a very different thing. Provided he jumped out far enough he would be sure to clear the propeller.

Mr Botibol advanced slowly to a position at the rail about twenty yards from the woman. She wasn't looking at him now. So much the better. He didn't want her watching him as he jumped off. So long as no-one was watching he would be able to say afterwards that he had slipped and fallen by accident. He peered over the side of the ship. It was a long, long drop. Come to think of it now, he might easily hurt himself badly if he hit the water flat. Wasn't there someone who once split his stomach open that way, doing a belly flop from the high dive? He must jump straight and land feet first. Go in like a knife. Yes, sir. The water seemed cold and deep and grey and it made him shiver to look at it. But it was now or never. Be a man, William Botibol, be a man. All right then . . . now . . . here goes . . .

He climbed up onto the wide wooden toprail, stood there poised, balancing for three terrifying seconds, then he leaped—he leaped up and out as far as he could go and at the same time he shouted, '*Help*!'

'*Help*! *Help*!' he shouted as he fell. Then he hit the water and went under.

When the first shout for help sounded, the woman who was leaning on the rail started up and gave a little jump of surprise. She looked around quickly and saw sailing past her through the air this small man dressed in white shorts and tennis-shoes, spreadeagled and shouting as he went. For a moment she looked as though she weren't quite sure what she ought to do: throw a lifebelt, run away and give the alarm, or simply turn and yell. She drew back a pace from the rail and swung half around facing up to the bridge, and for this brief moment she remained motionless, tense, undecided. Then almost at once she seemed to relax, and she leaned forward far over the rail, staring at the water where it was turbulent in the ship's wake. Soon a tiny round black head appeared in the foam, an arm was raised above it, once, twice, vigorously waving, and a small, faraway voice was heard calling something that was difficult to understand. The woman leaned still farther over the rail, trying to keep the little bobbing black speck in sight, but soon, so very soon, it was such a long way away that she couldn't even be sure it was there at all.

After a while another woman came out on deck. This one was bony and angular, and she wore horn-rimmed spectacles. She spotted the first woman and walked over to her, treading the deck in the deliberate, military fashion of all spinsters.

'So *there* you are,' she said.

The woman with the fat ankles turned and looked at her, but said nothing.

'I've been looking for you,' the bony one continued. 'Looking all over.'

'It's very odd,' the woman with the fat ankles said. 'A man dived overboard just now, with his clothes on.'

'Nonsense.'

'Oh yes. He said he wanted to get some exercise and he dived in and didn't even bother to take his clothes off.'

'You'd better come down now,' the bony woman said. Her mouth had suddenly become firm, her whole face sharp and alert, and she spoke less kindly than before. 'And don't you ever go wandering about on deck alone like this again. You know quite well you're meant to wait for me.'

'Yes, Maggie,' the woman with the fat ankles answered, and again she smiled, a tender trusting smile, and she took the hand of the other one and allowed herself to be led away across the deck.

'Such a nice man,' she said. 'He waved to me.'

My Oedipus Complex

by Frank O'Connor

Father was in the army all through the war—the First War, I mean—so up to the age of five I never saw much of him, and what I saw did not worry me. Sometimes I woke and there was a big figure in khaki peering down at me in the candlelight. Sometimes in the early morning I heard the slamming of the front door and the clatter of nailed boots down the cobbles of the lane. These were father's entrances and exits. Like Santa Claus he came and went mysteriously.

In fact, I rather liked his visits, though it was an uncomfortable squeeze between mother and him when I got into the big bed in the early morning. He smoked, which gave him a pleasant musty smell, and shaved, an operation of astounding interest. Each time he left a trail of souvenirs—model tanks and Gurkha knives with handles made of bullet cases, and German helmets and cap badges and button-sticks, and all sorts of military equipment—carefully stowed away in a long box on top of the wardrobe, in case they ever came in handy. There was a bit of the magpie about father; he expected everything to come in handy. When his back was turned, mother let me get a chair and rummage through his treasures. She didn't seem to think so highly of them as he did.

The war was the most peaceful period of my life. The window of my attic faced south-east. My mother had curtained it, but that had small effect. I always woke with the first light and, with all the responsibilities of the previous day melted, felt rather like the sun, ready to illumine and rejoice. Life never seemed so simple and clear and full of possibilities as then. I put my feet out from under the clothes—I called them Mrs Left and Mrs Right—and invented dramatic situations for them in which they discussed the problems of the day. At least Mrs Right did: she was very demonstrative; but I hadn't the same control of Mrs Left, so she mostly contented herself with nodding agreement.

They discussed what mother and I should do during the day, what Santa Claus should give a fellow for Christmas, and what steps should be taken to brighten the home. There was that little matter of the baby, for instance. Mother and I could never agree about that. Ours was the only house in the terrace without a new baby, and mother said we couldn't afford one till father came back from the war because they cost seventeen and six. That showed how simple she was. The Geneys up the road had a baby, and everyone knew they couldn't afford seventeen and six. It was probably a cheap baby, and mother wanted something really good, but I felt she was too exclusive. The Geneys' baby would have done us fine.

Having settled my plans for the day, I got up, put a chair under the attic window, and lifted the frame high enough to stick out my head. The window overlooked the front gardens of the terrace behind ours, and beyond these it looked over a deep valley to the tall red-brick houses terraced up the opposite hillside, which were all still in shadow, while those at our side of the valley were all lit up, though with long strange shadows that made them seem unfamiliar: rigid and painted.

After that I went into mother's room and climbed into the big bed. She woke and I began to tell her of my schemes. By this time, though I never seem to have noticed it, I was petrified in my nightshirt, and I thawed as I talked until, the last frost melted, I fell asleep beside her and woke again only when I heard her below in the kitchen making the breakfast.

After breakfast we went into town; heard Mass at St Augustine's and said a prayer for father, and did the shopping. If the afternoon was fine we either went for a walk in the country or paid a visit to mother's great friend in the convent, Mother St Dominic. Mother had them all praying for father, and every night, going to bed, I asked God to send him back safe from the war to us. Little, indeed, did I know what I was praying for!

One morning I got into the big bed, and there, sure enough, was father in his usual Santa Claus manner, but later instead of uniform he put on his best blue suit, and mother was as pleased as anything. I saw nothing to be pleased about, because, out of uniform, father was altogether less interesting, but she only beamed, and explained that our prayers had been answered, and off we went to Mass to thank God for having brought father safely home.

The irony of it! That very day when he came in to dinner he took off his boots and put on his slippers, donned the dirty old cap he wore about the house to save him from colds, crossed his legs, and began to talk gravely to mother, who looked anxious. Naturally, I disliked her looking anxious because it destroyed her good looks, so I interrupted him.

'Just a moment, Larry!' she said gently.

This was only what she said when we had boring visitors, so I attached no importance to it and went on talking.

'Do be quiet, Larry!' she said impatiently. 'Don't you hear me talking to Daddy?'

This was the first time I had heard those ominous words, 'talking to Daddy', and I couldn't help feeling that if this was how God answered prayers, he couldn't listen to them very attentively.

'Why are you talking to Daddy?' I asked with as great a show of indifference as I could muster.

'Because Daddy and I have business to discuss. Now don't interrupt again!'

In the afternoon, at mother's request, father took me for a walk. This time we went into town instead of out to the country, and I thought at first, in my usual optimistic way, that it might be an improvement. It was nothing of the sort. Father and I had quite different notions of a walk in town. He had no proper interest in trains, ships, and horses, and the only thing that seemed to divert him was talking to fellows as old as himself. When *I* wanted to stop he simply went on, dragging me behind him by the hand; when *he* wanted to stop I had no alternative but to do the same. I noticed that it seemed to be a sign that he wanted to stop for a long time whenever he leaned against a wall. The second time I saw him do it I got wild. He seemed to be settling himself forever. I pulled him by the coat and trousers, but unlike mother who, if you were too persistent, got into a wax and said: 'Larry, if you don't behave yourself, I'll give you a good slap,' father had an extraordinary capacity for amiable inattention. I sized him up and wondered would I cry, but he seemed to be too remote to be annoyed even by that. Really, it was like going for a walk with a mountain! He either ignored the wrenching and pummelling entirely, or else glanced down with a grin of amusement from his peak. I had never met anyone so absorbed in himself as he seemed.

At teatime, 'talking to Daddy' began again, complicated this time by the fact that he had an evening paper, and every few minutes he put it down and told mother something new out of it.

I felt this was foul play. Man for man, I was prepared to compete with him any time for mother's attention, but when he had it all made up for him by other people it left me no chance. Several times I tried to change the subject without success.

'You must be quiet while Daddy is reading, Larry,' mother said impatiently.

It was clear that she either genuinely liked talking to father better than talking to me, or else that he had some terrible hold on her which made her afraid to admit the truth.

'Mummy,' I said that night when she was tucking me up, 'do you think if I prayed hard God would send Daddy back to the war?'

She seemed to think about that for a moment.

'No, dear,' she said with a smile. 'I don't think he would.'

'Why wouldn't he, Mummy?'

'Because there isn't a war any longer, dear.'

'But, Mummy, couldn't God make another war, if He liked?'

'He wouldn't like to, dear. It's not God who makes wars, but bad people.'

'Oh!' I said.

I was disappointed about that. I began to think that God wasn't quite what he was cracked up to be.

Next morning I woke at my usual hour, feeling like a bottle of champagne. I put out my feet and invented a long conversation in which Mrs Right talked of the trouble she had with her own father till she put him in the Home. I didn't quite know what the Home was but it sounded the right place for father. Then I got my chair and stuck my head out of the attic window. Dawn was just breaking, with a guilty air that made me feel I had caught it in the act. My head bursting with stories and schemes, I stumbled in next door, and in the half-darkness scrambled into the big bed. There was no room at mother's side to I had to get between her and father. For the time being I had forgotten about him, and for several minutes I sat bolt upright, racking my brains to know what I could do with him. He was taking up more than his fair share of the bed, and I couldn't get comfortable, so I gave him several kicks that made him grunt and stretch. He made room all right, though. Mother waked and felt for me. I settled back comfortably in the warmth of the bed with my thumb in my mouth.

'Mummy!' I hummed, loudly and contentedly.

'Sssh! dear,' she whispered. 'Don't wake Daddy!'

This was a new development, which threatened to be even more serious than 'talking to Daddy'. Life without my early-morning conferences was unthinkable.

'Why?' I asked severely.

'Because poor Daddy is tired.'

This seemed to me a quite inadequate reason, and I was sickened by the sentimentality of her 'poor Daddy'. I never liked that sort of gush: it always struck me as insincere.

'Oh!' I said lightly. Then in my most winning tone: 'Do you know where I want to go with you today, Mummy?'

'No, dear,' she sighed.

'I want to go down the Glen and fish for thornybacks with my new net, and then I want to go out to the Fox and Hounds, and—'

'Don't-wake-Daddy!' she hissed angrily, clapping her hand across my mouth.

But it was too late. He was awake, or nearly so. He grunted and reached for the matches. Then he stared incredulously at his watch.

'Like a cup of tea, dear?' asked mother in a meek, hushed voice I had never heard her use before. It sounded almost as though she were afraid.

'Tea?' he exclaimed indignantly. 'Do you know what the time is?'

'And after that I want to go up the Rathcooney Road,' I said loudly, afraid I'd forget something in all those interruptions.

'Go to sleep at once, Larry!' she said sharply.

I began to snivel. I couldn't concentrate, the way that pair went on, and smothering my early-morning schemes was like burying a family from the cradle.

Father said nothing, but lit his pipe and sucked it, looking out into the shadows without minding mother or me. I knew he was mad. Every time I made a remark mother hushed me irritably. I was mortified. I felt it wasn't fair; there was even something sinister in it. Every time I had pointed out to her the waste of making two beds when we could both sleep in one, she had told me it was healthier like that, and now here was this man, this stranger, sleeping with her without the least regard for her health!

He got up early and made tea, but though he brought mother a cup he brought none for me.

'Mummy,' I shouted. 'I want a cup of tea, too.'

'Yes, dear,' she said patiently. 'You can drink from Mummy's saucer.'

That settled it. Either father or I would have to leave the house. I didn't want to drink from mother's saucer; I wanted to be treated as an equal in my own home, so just to spite her, I drank it all and left none for her. She took that quietly, too.

But that night when she was putting me to bed she said gently:

'Larry, I want you to promise me something.'

'What is it?' I asked.

'Not to come in and disturb poor Daddy in the morning. Promise?'

'Poor Daddy' again! I was becoming suspicious of everything involving that quite impossible man.

'Why?' I asked.

'Because poor Daddy is worried and tired and he doesn't sleep well.'

'Why doesn't he, Mummy?'

'Well, you know, don't you, that while he was at the war Mummy got the pennies from the Post Office?'

'From Miss MacCarthy?'

'That's right. But now, you see, Miss MacCarthy hasn't any more pennies, so Daddy must go out and find us some. You know what would happen if he couldn't?'

'No,' I said, 'tell us.'

'Well, I think we might have to go out and beg for them like the poor old woman on Fridays. We wouldn't like that, would we?'

'No,' I agreed. 'We wouldn't.'

'So you'll promise not to come in and wake him?'

'Promise.'

Mind you, I meant that. I knew pennies were a serious matter, and I was all against having to go out and beg like the old woman on Fridays. Mother laid out all my toys in a complete ring round the bed so that, whatever way I got out, I was bound to fall over one of them.

When I woke I remembered my promise all right. I got up and sat on the floor and played—for hours, it seemed to me. Then I got my chair and looked out of the attic window for more hours. I wished it was time for father to wake; I wished someone would make me a cup of tea. I didn't feel in the least like the sun; instead

I was bored and so very, very cold! I simply longed for the warmth and depth of the big featherbed.

At last I could stand it no longer. I went into the next room. As there was still no room at mother's side I climbed over her and she woke with a start.

'Larry,' she whispered, gripping my arm very tightly, 'what did you promise?'

'But I did, Mummy,' I wailed, caught in the very act. 'I was quiet for ever so long.'

'Oh dear, and you're perished!' she said sadly, feeling me all over. 'Now, if I let you stay will you promise not to talk?'

'But I want to talk, Mummy,' I wailed.

'That has nothing to do with it,' she said with a firmness that was new to me. 'Daddy wants to sleep. Now, do you understand that?'

I understood it only too well. I wanted to talk, he wanted to sleep—whose house was it, anyway?

'Mummy,' I said with equal firmness, 'I think it would be healthier for Daddy to sleep in his own bed.'

That seemed to stagger her, because she said nothing for a while.

'Now, once for all,' she went on, 'you're to be perfectly quiet or go back to your own bed. Which is it to be?'

The injustice of it got me down. I had convicted her out of her own mouth of inconsistency and unreasonableness, and she hadn't even attempted to reply. Full of spite, I gave father a kick, which she didn't notice but which made him grunt and open his eyes in alarm.

'What time is it?' he asked in a panic-stricken voice, not looking at mother but at the door, as if he saw someone there.

'It's early yet,' she replied soothingly. 'It's only the child. Go to sleep again . . . Now, Larry,' she added, getting out of bed, 'you've wakened Daddy and you must go back.'

This time, for all her quiet air, I knew she meant it, and knew that my principal rights and privileges were as good as lost unless I asserted them at once. As she lifted me, I gave a screech, enough to wake the dead, not to mind father. He groaned.

'That damn child! Doesn't he ever sleep?'

'It's only a habit, dear,' she said quietly, though I could see she was vexed.

'Well, it's time he got out of it,' shouted father, beginning to heave in the bed. He suddenly gathered all the bedclothes about him, turned to the wall, and then looked back over his shoulder with nothing showing only two small, spiteful, dark eyes. The man looked very wicked.

To open the bedroom door, mother had to let me down, and I broke free and dashed for the farthest corner, screeching. Father sat bolt upright in bed.

'Shut up, you little puppy!' he said in a choking voice.

I was so astonished that I stopped screeching. Never, never had anyone spoken to me in that tone before. I looked at him incredulously and saw his face convulsed with rage. It was only then that I fully realized how God had codded me, listening to my prayers for the safe return of this monster.

'Shut up, you!' I bawled, beside myself.

'What's that you said?' shouted father, making a wild leap out of the bed.

'Mick, Mick!' cried mother. 'Don't you see the child isn't used to you?'

'I see he's better fed than taught,' snarled father, waving his arms wildly. 'He wants his bottom smacked.'

All his previous shouting was as nothing to these obscene words referring to my person. They really made my blood boil.

'Smack your own!' I screamed hysterically. 'Smack you own! Shut up! Shut up!'

At this he lost his patience and let fly at me. He did it with the lack of conviction you'd expect of a man under mother's horrified eyes, and it ended up as a mere tap, but the sheer indignity of being struck at all by a stranger, a total stranger who had cajoled his way back from the war into our big bed as a result of my innocent intercession, made me completely dotty. I shrieked and shrieked, and danced in my bare feet, and father, looking awkward and hairy in nothing but a short grey army shirt, glared down at me like a mountain out for murder. I think it must have been then that I realized he was jealous too. And there stood mother in her nightdress, looking as if her heart was broken between us. I hoped she felt as she looked. It seemed to me that she deserved it all.

From that morning out my life was a hell. Father and I were enemies, open and avowed. We conducted a series of skirmishes against one another, he trying to steal my time with mother and I his. When she was sitting on my bed, telling me a story, he took to looking for some pair of old boots which he alleged he had left behind him at the beginning of the war. While he talked to mother I played loudly with my toys to show my total lack of concern. He created a terrible scene one evening when he came in from work and found me at his box, playing with his regimental badges, Gurkha knives, and button-sticks. Mother got up and took the box from me.

'You mustn't play with Daddy's toys unless he lets you, Larry,' she said severely. 'Daddy doesn't play with yours.'

For some reason father looked at her as if she had struck him and then turned away with a scowl.

'Those are not toys,' he growled, taking down the box again to see if I had lifted anything. 'Some of those curios are very rare and valuable.'

But as time went on I saw more and more how he managed to alienate mother and me. What made it worse was that I couldn't grasp his method or see what attraction he had for mother. In every possible way he was less winning than I. He had a common accent and made noises at his tea. I thought for a while that it might be the newspapers she was interested in, so I made up bits of news of my own to read to her. Then I thought it might be the smoking, which I personally thought attractive, and took his pipes and went round the house dribbling into them till he caught me. I even made noises at my tea, but mother only told me I was disgusting. It all seemed to hinge round that unhealthy habit of sleeping together, so I made a point of dropping into their bedroom and nosing round, talking to myself so that they wouldn't know I was watching them, but they were never up to anything that I could see. In the end it beat me. It seemed to depend on being grown-up and giving people rings, and I realized I'd have to wait.

But at the same time I wanted him to see that I was only waiting, not giving up the fight. One evening when he was being particularly obnoxious, chattering away well above my head, I let him have it.

'Mummy,' I said, 'do you know what I'm going to do when I grow up?'

'No, dear,' she replied, 'What?'

'I'm going to marry you,' I said quietly.

Father gave a great guffaw, but he didn't take me in. I knew it must only be pretence. And mother, in spite of everything, was pleased. I felt she was probably relieved to know that one day father's hold on her would be broken.

'Won't that be nice?' she said with a smile.

'It'll be very nice,' I said confidently. 'Because we're going to have lots and lots of babies.'

'That's right, dear,' she said placidly. 'I think we'll have one soon, and then you'll have plenty of company.'

I was no end pleased about that because it showed that in spite of the way she gave in to father she still considered my wishes. Besides, it would put the Geneys in their place.

It didn't turn out like that, though. To begin with, she was very preoccupied—I supposed about where she would get the seventeen and six—and though father took to staying out late in the evenings it did me no particular good. She stopped taking me for walks, became as touchy as blazes, and smacked me for nothing at all. Sometimes I wished I'd never mentioned the confounded baby—I seemed to have a genius for bringing calamity on myself.

And calamity it was! Sonny arrived in the most appalling hullabaloo—even that much he couldn't do without a fuss—and from the first moment I disliked him. He was a difficult child—so far as I was concerned he was always difficult—and demanded far too much attention. Mother was simply silly about him, and couldn't see when he was only showing off. As company he was worse than useless. He slept all day, and I had to go round the house on tiptoe to avoid waking him. It wasn't any longer a question of not waking father. The slogan now was 'Don't-wake-Sonny!' I couldn't understand why the child wouldn't sleep at the proper time, so whenever mother's back was turned I woke him. Sometimes to keep him awake I pinched him as well. Mother caught me at it one day and gave me a most unmerciful flaking.

One evening, when father was coming in from work, I was playing trains in the front garden. I let on not to notice him; instead, I pretended to be talking to myself, and said in a loud voice: 'If another bloody baby comes into this house, I'm going out.'

Father stopped dead and looked at me over his shoulder.

'What's that you said?' he asked sternly.

'I was only talking to myself,' I replied, trying to conceal my panic. 'It's private.'

He turned and went in without a word. Mind you, I intended it as a solemn warning, but its effect was quite different. Father started being quite nice to me. I could understand that, of course. Mother was quite sickening about Sonny. Even at mealtimes she'd get up and gawk at him in the cradle with an idiotic smile, and tell father to do the same. He was always polite about it, but he looked so puzzled you could see he didn't know what she was talking about. He complained of the way Sonny cried at night, but she only got cross and said that Sonny never cried except when there was something up with him—which was a flaming lie, because Sonny never had anything up with him, and only cried for attention. It was really painful to see how simple-minded she was. Father wasn't attractive, but he had a fine intelligence. He saw through Sonny, and now he knew that I saw through him as well.

One night I woke with a start. There was someone beside me in the bed. For one wild moment I felt sure it must be mother, having come to her senses and left father for good, but then I heard Sonny in convulsions in the next room, and mother saying: 'There! There! There!' and I knew it wasn't she. It was father. He was lying beside me, wide awake, breathing hard and apparently as mad as hell.

After a while it came to me what he was mad about. It was his turn now. After turning me out of the big bed, he had been turned out himself. Mother had no consideration now for anyone but that poisonous pup, Sonny. I couldn't help feeling sorry for father. I had been through it all myself, and even at that age I was magnanimous. I began to stroke him down and say: 'There! There!' He wasn't exactly responsive.

'Aren't you asleep either?' he snarled.

'Ah, come on and put your arm around us, can't you?' I said, and he did, in a sort of way. Gingerly, I suppose, is how you'd describe it. He was very bony but better than nothing.

At Christmas he went out of his way to buy me a really nice model railway.

Notes

CHARLES

8 *recess*: break; playtime

HOARSE CHESTNUTS

13 *mêlée*: confusion

MANHOOD

26 *Lilliputian rituals*: narrow, petty little people following a set pattern of behaviour, like those in the imaginary country of Lilliput in *Gulliver's Travels*

LADY OF THE ICE

29 *pirouette*: whirl on one foot

arabesque: when the body is bent forward on one leg with the corresponding arm outstretched and the other leg and arm extended horizontally backwards

30 *brilliants*: diamonds of especial brilliance, but these would be a synthetic variety

34 *myriad*: countless thousands

LITTLE OLD LADY FROM CRICKET CREEK

35 *performance evaluations*: judgements of people's work

Whistler's mother: term for an old woman, derived from a painting by James Whistler

38 *manila*: strong, light-brown paper that comes from Manila in the Philippines

THE SECRET LIFE OF WALTER MITTY

40 *obstreosis, streptothricosis, coreopsis*: real and fanciful terms for diseases

tertiary: in the third degree (an advanced stage)

intern: medical school graduate who is gaining practical experience by serving in a hospital

41 *craven*: cowardly; fearful

Notes

41 *carborundum*: substance used for polishing and scouring
42 *A & P*: Atlantic and Pacific (a supermarket)
43 *Archies*: anti-aircraft guns
Von Richtman's circus: planes commanded by an ace enemy flier
Saulier: imagined scene of the conflict
box barrage: anti-aircraft fire on three sides of an enemy
Auprès de Ma Blonde: a song: 'Close to my Blonde'
drugstore: chemist's shop that also sells general goods

THE RUUM

45 *interstellar overdrive*: a special high-speed gear for travelling between the stars.
Rigel: bright star in the constellation of Orion
the age of reptiles: the story starts during the age of reptiles, when a visiting spaceship leaves a 'ruum' on the earth by mistake. The ship is later destroyed in a space battle. The time then moves to the present, and Jim Irwin, a uranium prospector, lands in the valley where the ruum has been for the past few million years.
46 *cached*: concealed; stored away
Geiger counter: instrument for detecting radio-activity
47 *cougar*: panther or leopard
stegosaur: type of dinosaur with two rows of bony discs along its back
48 *saurian*: reptile such as a dinosaur, crocodile or lizard
tyrannosaurus: very large dinosaur (Tyrannosaurus Rex)
51 *pemmican*: dried meat, often mixed with other foods and used for emergency rations
54 *devil's mixture*: using anything available to create a violent explosion
55 *feral*: ferocious, like a beast of prey
57 *whirlybird*: helicopter
four-place job: 4-seater

A MAN CALLED HORSE

68 *coup stick*: stick similar to a truncheon, used for dealing a blow in warfare
69 *tepee*: conical tent used by the American Indians

Notes

71 *travois*: type of sledge
fall: autumn
74 *bedizened*: decorated in a gaudy manner
75 *coulee*: ravine or narrow valley

NATUK

93 *martens; mink*: small weasel-like animals valued for their fur
95 *Dogrib Indian*: Indian from the Dogrib tribes of north-western Canada
101 *coup de grâce*: death blow

DIP IN THE POOL

102 *purser*: officer who looks after the accounts on board ship
turbot: large tasty flatfish
hollandaise: sauce made from butter, egg-yolks and lemon-juice. It originally came from Holland
103 *auction pool*: on long sea journeys passengers often place bets on the distance the ship will travel in 24 hours. The captain first estimates the day's run according to weather conditions. Bids are then made for a range of numbers both below and above his estimate. The nearest correct estimate wins the 'pool', *ie* the total money
109 *bollard*: post used for securing ropes

MY OEDIPUS COMPLEX

115 *got into a wax*: became angry
121 *button-stick*: strip of wood or metal that is placed under brass buttons to enable them to be cleaned without soiling the cloth.

Teacher's Note

Reading Aloud

The stories are usually best enjoyed when read aloud. The reading should be strong and uninterrupted, bringing out where necessary the dialectal flavour. Difficult vocabulary should be simplified (*eg* by substituting 'unwise ' for 'injudicious' in *The Ruum*) and technical terms should be explained without breaking the flow of the story. Obscure references are explained in the Notes and can be jotted down in the teacher's copy before the lesson.

Discussion

This need not follow immediately, but after a short cathartic pause. If the story has had a strong emotional impact it is sometimes better to leave discussion until the following day, although in one or two instances the meaning will have to be elucidated. Each story should be read at one sitting, and where discussion is not required, as with *Hoarse Chestnuts,* timed to coincide with the end of the lesson. A page takes about 2–2½ minutes to read aloud.

Written work

Pupils should not be asked to write slavish summaries of the stories, nor to perform a critical autopsy on each. A better method is to ask for the *occasional* résumé or imaginative story based on the pupil's experience. It is also preferable at this level to omit any discussion of form or technique, but to regard the story primarily as a vehicle of meaning with a bearing on life. This volume is intended for use with *Excellence in English* Book 2 (Hodder & Stoughton) and follow-up exercises can be found there.

Acknowledgments

The author and publishers would like to thank the following for kindly granting permission for the reuse of copyright material in this book: the publishers of *Blackwood's Magazine* for 'Natuk' by George Bruce; Curtis Brown Ltd for 'Through the Tunnel' from *The Habit of Loving* by Doris Lessing and for 'Manhood' from *Death of the Hind Legs* by John Wain; Roald Dahl, Michael Joseph Ltd and Penguin Books Ltd for 'Dip in the Pool' from *Someone Like You*, © 1952 by Roald Dahl, and Copyright 1952 by Roald Dahl, reprinted from *Someone Like You*, by Roald Dahl, by permission of Alfred A. Knopf, Inc. (this story first appeared in *The New Yorker*); the Estate of the late Shirley Jackson for 'Charles' from *The Lottery and Other Stories*; Dorothy M Johnson and André Deutsch Ltd for 'A Man Called Horse' from *Indian Country* (1960); Sheila Markowitz for 'Lady of the Ice'; Frank O'Connor and Hamish Hamilton Ltd for 'My Oedipus Complex' from *Domestic Relations*; James Thurber and Hamish Hamilton Ltd for 'The Secret Life of Walter Mitty' from *The Vintage Thurber*, © the collection copyright Hamish Hamilton, London; also Mrs Helen Thurber, copyright © 1942 James Thurber, copyright © 1970 Helen Thurber, from *My World – And Welcome To It*, published by Harcourt Brace Jovanovich (originally printed in *The New Yorker*); 'Uneasy Homecoming' is reprinted by permission of A D Peters & Co Ltd and of Harold Matson Company, Inc., copyright © by Will F Jenkins; 'Little Old Lady from Cricket Creek', copyright © 1973 by Len Gray, is reprinted by permission of the author and the author's agents, Scott Meredith Literary Agency Inc, 845 Third Avenue, New York, NY 10022, USA.

In the case of 'The Ruum' it has not proved possible to trace the copyright owners, but full acknowledgment will be made in later printings if the publishers are notified as to whom they should contact.